Vascular Surgery
for the
House Officer

Second Edition

Vascular Surgery
for the
House Officer

Second Edition

Jon R. Cohen, M.D.

Chief of Vascular Surgery
Long Island Jewish Medical Center
Associate Professor of Surgery
Albert Einstein College of Medicine

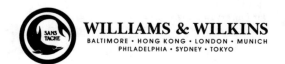

WILLIAMS & WILKINS
BALTIMORE · HONG KONG · LONDON · MUNICH
PHILADELPHIA · SYDNEY · TOKYO

Editor: Michael G. Fisher
Associate Editor: Fran Witthauer
Copy Editor: Anne Schwartz
Designer: Dan Pfisterer
Production Coordinator: Adèle Boyd-Lanham

Copyright © 1992
Williams & Wilkins
428 East Preston Street
Baltimore, Maryland 21202, USA

Accurate indications, adverse reactions, and dosage schedules for drugs are provided in this book, but it is possible that they may change. The reader is urged to review the package information data of the manufacturers of the medications mentioned.

Printed in the United States of America

First Edition 1986

Library of Congress Cataloging in Publication Data

Cohen, Jon R.
  Vascular surgery for the house officer / Jon R. Cohen. — 2nd ed.
    p.   cm.
  Includes bibliographical references and index.
  ISBN 0-683-02052-8
  1. Blood-vessels—Surgery—Handbooks, manuals, etc. I. Title. [DNLM: 1. Vascular Surgery—handbooks. WG 39 C678v]
RD598.5.C6   1992   617'.413—dc20
DNLM/DLC   91-24507
for Library of Congress   CIP

91   92   93   94   95
1   2   3   4   5   6   7   8   9   10

To my parents, Mickey and Sylvia, for making it all possible

and

To my wife, Karen and my daughter Leslie, for keeping it all so wonderful.

The first edition of <u>Vascular Surgery for the House Officer</u> was published in 1986 and has sold approximately 15,000 copies. The book originally grew out of a need for a concise basic fund of knowledge of vascular surgery which would be readily available to the medical student, resident and nonspecialist. The second edition updates the first edition, in addition to adding several new chapters including a chapter on Vascular Trauma, a chapter on Portal Hypertension, and a chapter on Alternate Techniques for the Treatment of Vascular Occlusive Disease. I hope that these new chapters add more depth to the book and that the update will keep it current.

Once again, this book is by no means a complete textbook of vascular surgery or an atlas of how to do vascular operations. Its purpose is to provide a core of medical information that needs to be known by any medical student or physician regardless of his or her specialty and a guide for the junior house officer in the pre- and postoperative care of vascular patients, with some specific facts for quick review by senior residents. As in the first edition, drawings of some of the more important anatomical relationships are also included. In this second edition, we hope to achieve the practical needs of both the medical student and the house officer in the treatment of patients with vascular surgery problems.

Jon R. Cohen, M.D.

Acknowledgment

I would like to thank five surgeons who have had a profound affect on my life and training:

Karen M. Kostroff, M.D. (my wife)

John A. Mannick, M.D.

G. Tom Shires, M.D.

Malcolm O. Perry, M.D.

Leslie Wise, M.D.

Contents

Chapter 1

Evaluating the Patient with Vascular Disease

Peripheral vascular disease is only one manifestation of the multisystem effects of extensive atherosclerotic disease. When evaluating patients with specific vascular complaints, it is important to keep in mind that the majority of patients have coexistent cardiac and other vascular disease.

Of those patients undergoing major vascular reconstruction, preoperative evaluation reveals that:

-20% have had a previous myocardial infarction;

-7% have had previous congestive heart failure;

-4% have had a previous arrhythmia;

-60% have abnormal electrocardiograms;

-7% have had a previous cerebrovascular accident.

Specific cardiac evaluation with cardiac catheterization in 1000 patients with peripheral arterial disease at the Cleveland Clinic revealed that severe correctable coronary artery disease was found in:

-31% of those patients with abdominal aortic aneurysms;

-26% of those patients with cerebrovascular disease;

-21% of those patients with lower extremity ischemia.

1

Overall <u>30%</u> <u>of</u> <u>patients</u> presenting with vascular disease had <u>severe</u> <u>coronary</u> <u>artery</u> <u>disease</u>.

HISTORY

Manifestations

1. <u>INTERMITTENT</u> <u>CLAUDICATION</u> is ischemic muscle pain that occurs as a result of <u>inadequate</u> <u>blood</u> <u>flow</u> from proximal arterial lesions and occurs most frequently in the calf muscles. It is classically described as a <u>cramping</u> <u>pain</u> that occurs with exercise and is relieved within several minutes by rest. Commonly it is described as a tiredness or weakness especially within the thighs or buttocks. Because of collateral blood supply, two different levels of disease are usually required before claudication occurs, i.e., aortic and iliac disease for thigh/buttock claudication or femoral and popliteal disease for calf claudication. It is important to establish during each office visit how far, usually in city blocks, a patient can walk without getting the pain. A decrease in distance is usually a sign of progressive disease. Other common possibilities in the differential diagnosis of leg pain include sciatica, spinal stenosis, diabetic neuropathy, and osteoarthritis of the hip.

2. <u>REST</u> <u>PAIN</u> indicates more severe disease than claudication, as the pain is continuous from constant

insufficient blood supply. It occurs only in the <u>foot</u> and is classically described as a <u>burning pain in the forefoot aggravated by elevation.</u> The pain usually <u>occurs at night</u> when the patient is reclining and is relieved only when the patient gets up to walk around. The patient usually adapts by sleeping with his foot hanging over the edge of the bed.

3. <u>IMPOTENCE</u> is commonly associated with thigh and buttock claudication as a result of <u>aortoiliac insufficiency</u>. It can be seen with isolated hypogastric insufficiency and is manifest by the inability to achieve or maintain an effective erection.

4. <u>TIA</u> (<u>transient ischemic attack</u>) is a focal or generalized neurological dysfunction with transient symptoms that lasts for <u>less than 24 hours</u>. Common symptoms of focal attacks include speech, ocular, sensory, or motor disturbances of varying degrees. An episode of <u>transient monocular blindness</u> is called <u>amaurosis fugax</u>.

5. <u>PREVIOUS CARDIAC DISEASE</u> including angina, myocardial infarction, and arrhythmias as discussed above is important to establish.

<u>RISK FACTORS</u>

1. <u>SMOKING</u> is one of the most important contributing factors in the development of the majority of peripheral vascular disease. How many packs/day? How many years?

2. <u>DIABETICS</u> routinely have some degree of vascular disease. Juvenile or adult onset? Insulin controlled? How much?

3. <u>HYPERTENSION</u> is associated with cardiac disease and commonly found in patients with abdominal aortic aneurysms. How long has the patient been hypertensive? What medications?

4. <u>DEEP</u> <u>VENOUS</u> <u>THROMBOSIS</u> or <u>PULMONARY</u> <u>EMBOLUS</u> previously?

5. <u>HYPERLIPIDEMIAS</u> or known <u>CLOTTING</u> <u>ABNORMALITIES</u>?

<u>PHYSICAL EXAMINATION</u>

1. <u>PALPATION</u> <u>OF</u> <u>PULSES</u> carotid, radial, femoral, popliteal, dorsalis pedis, and posterior tibial pulses are mandatory in any physical examination. It is important to establish the quality of the vessels as well as the pulse volume when examining the pulse. In the femoral region the posterior plaque in a diseased vessel is usually palpable.

2. <u>BRUITS</u> over the carotid and femoral arteries are especially important to document in the routine physical as well as the presence of abdominal bruits.

3. <u>INSPECT</u> the extremities for pallor, cyanosis, rubor, ulceration, gangrene, atrophy, temperature, or varicosities. <u>Trophic</u> <u>changes</u> of peripheral vascular insufficiency include loss of hair, shiny skin, and thickened toenails.

4. <u>DOPPLER</u> measurement of the <u>ankle/brachial</u> <u>index</u> (Chapter 11) along with the blood pressure of each arm should be

recorded in every vascular patient.

LEG ULCERATION

Leg ulcerations are usually a result of ischemia, venous stasis disease, or neuropathy secondary to either diabetes or syphilis. The following are the important differences between these three types of ulceration:

	ISCHEMIC	STASIS	NEUROPATHIC
Pain	Severe	Mild	None
Location	Toes	Ankle	Heel or meta-tarsal head
Bleeding	Little	Venous ooze	Brisk
Associated findings	Trophic changes	Stasis dermatitis	Neuropathy

(From: Rutherford, R.B., Vascular Surgery, ed 1, Table 1-2, p 13, W.B. Saunders Co., Philadelphia, 1977.)

Figure 1.1. Important data to record for all vascular patients.

HISTORY

1. Cardiac disease? Angina? MI? Arrhythmia?

2. Claudication?   How far?   Rest pain?   Impotence?

3. TIA?   Stroke?

4. Smoking? How long? Packs/day?

5. Diabetes?   How long? Insulin?   How much?

6. Hypertension?   How long?   Meds?

7. Clotting abnormalities?   DVT?   Pulmonary embolus?

8. Hyperlipidemia?

PHYSICAL EXAM

1. Blood pressure: Right_____   Left _____

2. Pulses:

0-ABSENT, 1+ BARELY PALPABLE, 2+ NORMAL, 3+ ENLARGED,

4+ ANEURYSMAL:

CAROTID	RADIAL	FEMORAL	POPLITEAL	D. PEDIS	POST.TIB
Rt_____	_____	_____	_____	_____	_____
Lt_____	_____	_____	_____	_____	_____
BRUIT___	_____				

3. Cardiac exam?

4. Inspection of extremities: Perfusion?   Varicosities?
   Trophic changes?   Tissue loss?

5. Abdominal aortic aneurysm?

6. Ankle/brachial index: R   L

SUGGESTED READINGS

1. Barker, W.F.: Diagnostic Problems. In Peripheral Arterial Disease, ed 2, pp 75-101. W.B. Saunders Co., Philadelphia, 1975.

2. Cooperman, M., Pflug, M., Martin, E., et al.: Cardiovascular Risk Factors in Patients with Peripheral Vascular Disease. Surgery 84:505, 1978.

3. Hertzer, N.: Fatal Myocardial Infarction Following Abdominal Aortic Aneurysm Resection. Ann Surg 192:667, 1980.

4. Hertzer, N.: Fatal Myocardial Infarction Following Lower Extremity Revascularization. Ann Surg 193:492, 1981.

5. Hertzer, N., Bevin, E., Young, J., et al.: Coronary Artery Disease in Peripheral Vascular Patients. Ann Surg 199:223, 1984.

6. Hertzer, N., Lees, D.: Fatal Myocardial Infarction Following Carotid Endarterectomy. Ann Surg 194:212, 1981.

7. O'Donnell, T., Callow, A., Willet, C., et al.: The Impact of Coronary Artery Disease on Carotid Endarterectomy. Ann Surg 198:705, 1983.

8. Rutherford, R.B.: Initial Clinical Evaluation-The Vascular Consultation. In Vascular Surgery, edited by R.B. Rutherford, ed 1, pp 3-13. W.B. Saunders Co., Philadelphia, 1977.

Chapter 2

Drugs Commonly Used in Vascular Surgery

1. HEPARIN

Heparin is a naturally occurring mucopolysaccharide that is negatively charged, thereby complexing with positively charged plasma proteins. Heparin is extracted from the mast cells of different animal tissues (bovine lung or cattle and hog intestine), so the potency varies with the milligram weight. Final preparations are standardized according to biological activity and expressed as units of activity. It must be given I.V. or sub-Q, has a half-life of 1 1/2 hours, and is partially excreted in the urine. Heparin is monitored by its prolongation of the partial thromboplastin time (PTT).

Heparin interferes with the formation of fibrin by acting at three sites:

1. Slowing the conversion of prothrombin to thrombin (Fig. 2.1);

2. Potentiating the effect of antithrombin III; antithrombin III is a naturally occurring inhibitor of thrombin which acts as a co-factor with heparin to markedly reduce the effects of thrombin on fibrinogen (Fig. 2.1);

8

3. <u>Decreasing</u>   <u>platelet</u> <u>adhesiveness</u> by increasing the electronegative potential of the vessel wall (Fig. 2.1).

Heparin-induced <u>thrombocytopenia</u> is a well known complication of the drug. Heparin can be <u>neutralized</u> quickly with I.V. <u>protamine</u> <u>sulfate</u> at a dose of 1 mg of protamine sulfate for every 100 units of active heparin.

2. <u>COUMADIN</u>

Coumadin (sodium warfarin) is effective if given orally. It functions by <u>inhibiting the production of the vitamin K-dependent</u> <u>factors</u> of the coagulation cascade, II (prothrombin), VII, IX, and X (Fig. 2.1). Because of the long half-lives of several of the vitamin K-dependent factors, it may take as long as 3 days for anticoagulation to begin. The drug is metabolized by the <u>microsomal enzyme</u> <u>system</u> within the liver and is thereby affected by other drugs which either induce or inhibit these liver enzymes. The <u>half-life of Coumadin is 36 hours</u>, but it can take from 1 to 8 days for the prothrombin time to return to normal if the drug is discontinued. More rapid correction can be achieved with I.M. vitamin K and fresh frozen plasma. Coumadin is monitored by its prolongation of the prothrombin time (PT).

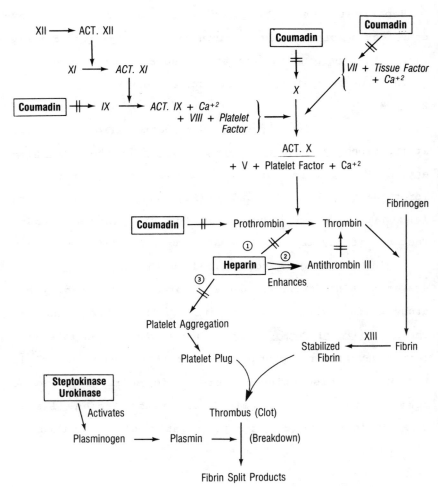

Figure 2.1.   The sites of inhibition by Coumadin, heparin, streptokinase and urokinase on the coagulation cascade.

ANTIPLATELET DRUGS

Aspirin and Persantine are antiplatelet drugs that work by affecting the prostaglandin pathways within platelets and endothelial cells. They are both monitored by their effects on the platelet plug-forming mechanism as measured by prolongation of the Ivy bleeding time.

Prostaglandins (PGs) are 20-carbon unsaturated fatty acids which act as important messengers for the control of cellular activity. In response to many different stimuli at the cell membrane level, phospholipase is activated to produce arachidonic acid from available phospholipids, thus initiating prostaglandin production (Fig. 2.2). Up to this point the pathway is similar within platelets and endothelial cells, but subsequently the end product differs. Within the endothelial cell the end product is prostacyclin (PGI-2), whereas within the platelet the end product is thromboxane A-2 (TXA-2) (Fig. 2.2).

PGI-2, mostly made by the endothelial cell, increases the intracellular levels of cAMP. cAMP then inhibits platelet aggregation and acts as a vasodilator (Fig. 2.2).

TXA-2, mostly made by the platelet, increases the levels of cGMP. cGMP then promotes platelet aggregation and causes vasoconstriction (Fig. 2.2).

The final result of the interaction between platelets and endothelial cells upon the vessel intima is a balance of the opposite effects of PGI-2 and TXA-2.

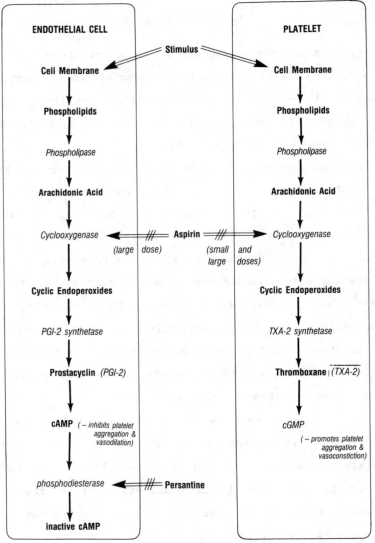

Figure 2.2.   The sites of inhibition of aspirin and Persantine on the prostaglandin pathway within the endothelial cell and platelet.

1. ASPIRIN

   Conventional doses of aspirin (325 mg/day) inhibit the entire prostaglandin pathway by irreversibly acetylating cyclooxygenase (Fig. 2.2). The result is the complete inhibition of PGI-2 and TXA-2 production. Since both of these prostaglandins have opposing effects on platelet aggregation and vascular tone, the net effect at this dosage is very small. Inhibition is permanent within the platelet but can be overcome within the endothelial cell in 1 to 2 days by the production of new cyclooxygenase.

   Small doses of aspirin (100 mg/day) have been found to selectively inhibit platelet cyclooxygenase more than endothelial cyclooxygenase, thereby increasing the relative amounts of prostacyclin and decreasing the amount of TXA-2 (Fig. 2.2). The resulting desired effect is a decrease in platelet aggregation in response to injury and vasodilation, thereby decreasing subsequent thrombosis in native arteries and vascular grafts.

2. PERSANTINE (dipyridamole)

   Persantine is a phosphodiesterase inhibitor which acts by inhibiting the breakdown of cAMP within platelets (Fig 2.2). The result is an increase in platelet cAMP which subsequently decreases platelet aggregation. Persantine used in conjunction with aspirin seems to have an enhanced effect.

THROMBOLYTIC AGENTS

Both streptokinase and urokinase are used for lysis of clots within the arterial and venous system. Both drugs are contraindicated in any setting of recent bleeding where clot lysis may be dangerous, i.e., recent surgery or gastrointestinal bleeding. During thrombolytic therapy the thrombin time should be prolonged 2-5 times the control value to confirm activation of the fibrolytic system. The thrombin time and hematocrit should be monitored every 6 to 12 hours during therapy.

1. STREPTOKINASE

This a nonenzymatic protein that is produced by group C beta-hemolytic streptococci. Streptokinase works by a two-step activation of plasminogen. Plasminogen then acts to cause the formation of the proteolytic enzyme plasmin which actively causes clot dissolution (Fig. 2.1). The usual dose is 250,000 IU loading dose and then 100,000 IU/hour for 24-72 hours.

2. UROKINASE

Urokinase is an enzymatic protein produced by human renal parenchymal cells grown in tissue culture and is much more expensive than streptokinase to produce. It activates plasminogen directly to produce plasmin (Fig. 2.1). The dosage is 4400 IU/kg loading dose and then 4400 IU/hour for 12 hours.

PENTOXIFYLLINE (Trental)

Pentoxifylline is used to treat patients with intermittent claudication by altering the rheology of red blood cells. It works to improve blood flow by increasing red cell flexibility, thus easing the passage of red cells through the microcirculation.

Pentoxifylline increases walking distance 25-40% in patients with claudication. Patients on placebo and a vigorous exercise program can increase their walking distance 20-30%; thus the actual advantage of the drug is very limited when compared to a good exercise program. The major disadvantage is that up to 30% of patients will have gastrointestinal side effects when taking the drug.

SUGGESTED READINGS

1. Bell, W., Meek, A.: Guidelines for the Use of Thrombolytic Agents. N Engl J Med 301:1266, 1979.

2. Chesebro, J., Clements, I., Fuster, M., et al.: A Platelet Inhibitor Drug Trial in Coronary Artery Bypass Operations. Benefits of Perioperative Dipyridamole and Aspirin Therapy on Early Postoperative Vein Graft Patency. N Engl J Med 307:73, 1982.

3. Dardik, H., Sussman, B., Kahn, M., et al.: Lysis of Arterial Clot by Intravenous or Intra-arterial Administration of Streptokinase. Surg Gynecol Obstet 158:137, 1984.

4. Jacobsen, D.: Prostaglandins and Cardiovascular Disease- A Review. <u>Surgery</u> 93:564, 1983.

5. McCann, R., Hagen, P., Fuchs, J.: Aspirin and Dipyridamole Decrease Intimal Hyperplasia in Experimental Vein Grafts. <u>Ann</u> <u>Surg</u> 191:238, 1980.

6. Nussbaum, M., Moschos, C.: Anticoagulants and Anticoagulation. <u>Med</u> <u>Clin</u> <u>North</u> <u>Am</u> 60:855, 1976.

7. Perry, M., Horton, J.: Kinetics of Heparin Administration. <u>Arch</u> <u>Surg</u> 111:403, 1976.

8. Porter, J.M., Cutler, B.S., Lee, B.Y., et al: Pentoxifylline Efficacy in the Treatment of Intermittent Claudication: Multicenter Controlled Double Blind Trial With Objective Assessment of Chronic Occlusive Arterial Disease Patients. <u>Am</u> <u>Heart</u> <u>J</u> 104:66-72, 1982.

9. Richter, R.: Antiplatelet Therapy in Surgery. <u>Infect</u> <u>Surg</u> p. 137 Feb 1984.

10. Silver, D., Kapsch, D., Tsoi, E.: Heparin Induced Thrombocytopenia, Thrombosis, and Hemorrhage. <u>Ann</u> <u>Surg</u> 198:301, 1983.

11. Van Breda, A., Robinson, J., Feldman, L., et al: Local Thrombolysis in the Treatment of Arterial Graft Occlusions. <u>J</u> <u>Vasc</u> <u>Surg</u> 1:103, 1984.

Chapter 3

Atherosclerosis

The majority of disease treated by vascular surgeons is a result of atherosclerosis. While the disease is always diffuse, large deposits usually occur segmentally throughout the vascular tree at predictable critical points. The lesions result in segmental obstruction which is frequently amenable to surgical intervention.

ARTERIAL ANATOMY

Muscular and elastic arteries are divided histologically into three layers (Fig. 3.1):

1. The INTIMA contains endothelial cells with occasional subendothelial smooth muscle cells in a single layer. It is separated from the media by the internal elastic membrane.

2. The MEDIA is the major structural support for the artery. It contains smooth muscle cells, collagen, elastin, and proteoglycans. The blood supply for the inner part of the media is from direct diffusion through the intima while the outer part of the media is supplied by smaller penetrating arteries known as vasa vasorum. The media is separated from the outermost layer, the adventitia, by the external elastic membrane.

3. The ADVENTITIA contains fibroblasts, collagen, and elastic tissue and is important for overall strength and structure.

17

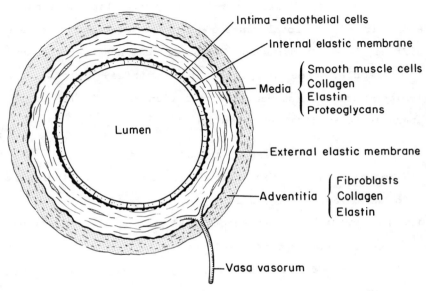

Figure 3.1.   Cross-section anatomy of an artery.

The primary event in the development of atherosclerosis is <u>injury</u> <u>to</u> <u>the</u> <u>endothelial</u> <u>cell</u>. Some of the more common inciting factors are

1. <u>Tobacco</u>- possibly a direct harmful effect of nicotine;
2. <u>Diabetes</u>- probably anoxia to the endothelial cell;
3. <u>Radiation</u>- probably anoxia or a direct harmful effect;
4. <u>Hypertension</u>- increased shearing forces on the endothelial cell;
5. <u>Hyperlipidemia</u>- abnormal endothelial cell metabolism;
6. <u>Direct</u> <u>arterial</u> <u>injury</u>- direct endothelial injury.

<u>Focal</u> lesions of atherosclerosis develop in areas more prone to constant endothelial injury such as <u>arterial</u> <u>bifurcations</u> or areas of <u>posterior</u> <u>fixation</u> where shearing forces and turbulent flow are highest. Common, predictable locations for the focal lesions include all of the aortic branches at their takeoff, the aortic bifurcation, the common iliac bifurcation, the common femoral bifurcation, the common carotid bifurcation, and the superficial femoral artery at Hunter's canal where it is fixed.

Atherosclerotic lesions of the <u>aorta</u> resulting in both occlusive and aneurysmal disease occur <u>most</u> <u>frequently</u> <u>in</u> <u>the</u> <u>abdomen</u> as compared to the thorax. This preferential distribution is probably a result of the <u>marked</u> <u>absence</u> <u>of</u> <u>vasa</u> <u>vasorum</u> <u>within</u> <u>the</u> <u>abdominal</u> <u>aorta</u> and the subsequent endothelial cell anoxia.

The endothelial cell response to the initial injury is a complex chain of events involving platelet metabolism, prostaglandin synthesis, smooth muscle cell proliferation, and cholesterol metabolism, all of which form the basis for the development of atherosclerotic lesions. The lesions that result are classified histologically into three groups:

1. FATTY STREAKS are the earliest lesion, appearing raised and yellow. Histologically, large amounts of cholesterol esters (lipid) are found within macrophages and smooth muscle cells.

2. FIBROUS PLAQUES are more advanced lesions containing large numbers of smooth muscle cells. The lesion extrudes into the arterial lumen and consists of a lipid covered by fibrous material.

3. COMPLICATED PLAQUES are the result of long-standing atherosclerosis when fibrous plaques become necrotic, ulcerated, and/or calcified.

The exact relationship between hyperlipidemia and atherosclerosis is still unknown, but a large body of evidence exists to strongly support a cause and effect relationship between plasma cholesterol, low density lipoproteins, and atherogenesis. Some of the evidence that implicates cholesterol in a primary role is

1. It is a major component of plaques and is derived from low density lipoproteins which accumulate in atheromatous lesions.

2. There is a strong epidemiological relationship between serum cholesterol and coronary heart disease.

3. Familial hyperlipidemia type II patients develop atherosclerosis at a much younger age.

4. Evidence exists that lowering serum cholesterol may help in regressing atherosclerotic lesions.

5. Increasing serum cholesterol in certain animal models increases the development of atherosclerotic lesions.

The important factors for further development of atherosclerosis to discuss and control in patients presenting with vascular disease or in those young patients with advanced disease are

1. HYPERLIPIDEMIA   5. PHYSICAL ACTIVITY

2. HYPERTENSION   6. OBESITY

3. CIGARETTE SMOKING   7. STRESS

4. DIABETES   8. FAMILIAL HISTORY

SUGGESTED READINGS

1. Barker, W.F.: Pathology and Pathogenesis. In Peripheral Arterial Disease, ed 2, pp 56-73. W.B. Saunders Co., Philadelphia, 1975.

2. Davignon, J.: The Lipid Hypothesis. Arch Surg 113:28, 1978.

3. Depalma, R., Clowes, A.: Interventions in Atherosclerosis: A Review for Surgeons. Surgery 84:175, 1978.

4. Fredrickson, D.: Atherosclerosis and Other Forms of atherosclerosis. In <u>Principles of Internal Medicine</u>, edited by G. Thorn et al., vol 8, pp 670-675, 1297-1307. McGraw-Hill, New York, 1977.

5. Margolis, S.: Management of Systemic Atheromatous Disease. In <u>Vascular Surgery</u>, edited by R.B. Rutherford, ed 1, pp 309-316, 488-489. W.B. Saunders Co., Philadelphia, 1977.

Chapter 4

Deep Venous Thrombosis (DVT) and Pulmonary Emboli (PE)

One of the most common and potentially life-threatening problems seen by the vascular surgeon is the diagnosis, prophylaxis, and treatment of DVT and/or PE in both medical and surgical patients. The magnitude of the problem is enormous, with a conservative estimate of 2.5 million cases of DVT/year, 600,000 cases of PE/year, and 200,000 deaths/year in the United States related to PE. In intensively studied postoperative patients, an estimated 30-40% will develop DVT; of autopsies where the leg veins are meticulously dissected, 50-60% of patients have DVT. It is important to realize that DVT/PE is a life-threatening disease and that those patients at higher risk should be identified and treated aggressively.

RISK FACTORS

The pathophysiology for the development of venous thrombosis is based upon those factors as originally described by Virchow's triad:

1. Trauma to the vein wall;

2. Venous stasis from decreased flow;

3. Increased blood coagulability.

Based upon these criteria, any patient with one of the following factors is at a higher risk for developing DVT. The relative risk as compared to the general population is given on the right hand side.

RISK INCREASE

1. PREGNANCY/POSTPARTUM: Increases stasis on the   5-6 x
    pelvic veins and increases clotting factors.

2. ESTROGENS: Birth control pills or estrogen   4-7 x
    chemotherapy has several effects, including
    decreasing vascular tone, venous stasis, and
    increasing clotting factors while decreasing
    antithrombin III levels.

3. PAST HISTORY: Patients with previous episodes   3-5 x
    of DVT have a very high rate of recurrence.

4. OBESITY: This is possibly due to a decrease in   2 x
    fibrinolytic activity.

5. CANCER: This may be due to associated factors   2-3 x
    such as prolonged bed rest, surgery, or heart
    disease.

6. PARALYSIS, PROLONGED BED REST, IMMOBILITY: Any   3 x
    situation where the patient is bedridden for
    prolonged periods, such as a stroke or
    paraplegia, increases the risk due to venous
    stasis.

7. HEMATOLOGICAL disease that cause increased
    coagulability or sludging, such as the

myeloproliferative disorders.

8. <u>TRAUMA</u> of any sort and especially direct injury to the lower extremity causes venous stasis from immobility and thrombosis from direct venous injury. Of those patients dying after a <u>hip</u> <u>fracture</u>, up to 50% die as a result of a PE.

9. <u>CARDIAC DISEASE</u> resulting in low cardiac   3-4 x output, immobilization, and especially arrhythmias is associated with a much higher incidence of both DVT and PE.

10. <u>AGE ≥ 40 YEARS</u> increases the risk, most likely as a result of the higher prevalence of heart disease and cancer in the older population.

11. <u>VARICOSE VEINS</u> increases the risk in patients undergoing surgery, which may reflect an associated valvular incompetence within the deep venous system and subsequent stasis.

12. <u>SURGERY</u> alone results in <u>venous stasis while the patient is on the operating room table</u>. The longer the operative procedure and the greater its magnitude, the higher the risk of DVT. Surgery in combination with any of the above risk factors markedly increases the risk of postoperative DVT and subsequent PE. In those patients undergoing major surgery the risk of thromboembolism is increased 50% with obesity and up to 300% with cardiac disease or

a past history of DVT.

OPERATIVE PROPHYLAXIS IN HIGH-RISK PATIENTS

Recognizing high-risk patients for preoperative prophylaxis is extremely important for two reasons:

1. It has been estimated that some 4000-8000 deaths/year could be prevented with the use of prophylactic low-dose heparin in higher risk patients undergoing surgery.

2. Pulmonary embolus is the most common cause of death following routine procedures such as cholecystectomy, herniorrhaphy, and hysterectomy.

The majority of venous thrombi are formed when the patient is on the operating table, so that effective prophylaxis needs to begin preoperatively. There have been many mechanical and pharmacological methods used for prophylaxis, but the two most effective methods used today are

1. LOW-DOSE HEPARIN (MINI-HEPARIN): Given at a dose of 5000 units sub-Q every 12 hours starting 2 hours preoperatively. This can reduce the incidence of DVT from 25% to 7%. The major problem has been bleeding complications at a rate of 0-27%. (See the discussion on the mechanism of action of heparin, Chapter 2.)

2. INTERMITTENT PNEUMATIC CALF COMPRESSION (IPCC): If applied during surgery and in the postoperative period, these devices are equally as effective as low-dose heparin but without the bleeding complications. The

biggest problem is <u>patient</u> <u>discomfort</u>. The effect is both mechanical by direct calf compression and chemical by inducing plasminogen activity and subsequent systemic fibrinolysis.

<u>THE</u> <u>PATIENT</u> <u>WITH</u> <u>DVT</u>

The most important factor for the diagnosis of DVT is a high index of suspicion and aggressive diagnostic testing in patients in the high-risk categories listed above. The clinical diagnosis of DVT based upon history and physical exam alone is poor, with only a 50% accuracy rate. Physical findings usually appear late, and at least 50% of DVT episodes are silent. When present, the most common findings are erythema, tenderness, and swelling of the calf, all of which can be easily confused with a variety of disorders. <u>Homans'</u> <u>sign</u> for DVT is tenderness in the calf muscles with dorsiflexion of the foot.

<u>PHLEGMASIA</u> <u>CERULEA</u> <u>DOLENS</u> is a severe form of <u>ileo-femoral</u> <u>venous</u> <u>thrombosis</u> resulting in massive swelling, pain, tenderness, and cyanosis of the entire involved extremity. <u>PHLEGMASIA</u> <u>ALBA</u> <u>DOLENS</u> (milk leg) is a variant of the severe thrombosis when the arterial supply is compromised as a result of the massive swelling and the leg becomes white in color.

Diagnostic testing is essential for DVT and includes the following methods:

1. <u>DOPPLER</u> <u>ULTRASOUND</u> works by the Doppler principle (Fig. 4.1). A sound wave is generated by the Doppler which bounces off nonmoving tissues unchanged. Moving particles (blood flow) will interrupt the returning sound wave and cause a change in frequency which is detected by the Doppler. The change in frequency of the returning wave is then converted into an audible signal.

Doppler ultrasound is an essential extension of the physical exam in evaluating patients for DVT. The exam includes listening for flow in the anterior tibial, posterior tibial, popliteal, and femoral veins. Venous flow is described as "howling or blowing sounds in a cave or tunnel" and is usually next to the arterial counterpart.

The essentials of the exam include:

    a. Listening for the presence of the signal as compared with the opposite side;

    b. <u>Augmentation</u> of flow with <u>expiration</u> and decrease in flow with <u>inspiration</u>;

    c. <u>Augmentation</u> of flow with <u>calf</u> <u>compression</u>.

The overall accuracy of the Doppler exam is 80-85%, but it depends largely upon the experience of the examiner. A normal exam is usually adequate to rule out femoral popliteal disease, but small thrombi within the soleal veins cannot be detected. An abnormal exam usually requires a second diagnostic test for confirmation before therapy is begun.

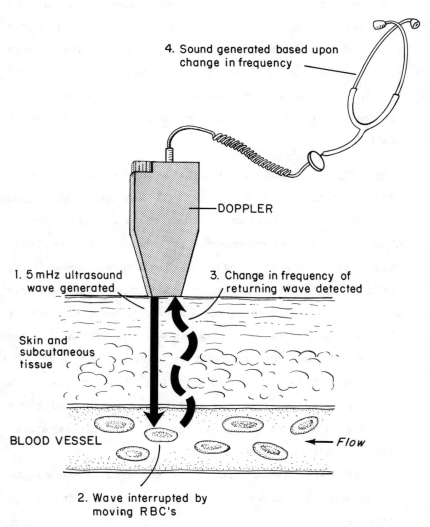

Figure 4.1. The Doppler principle in detecting blood flow.

2. <u>VENOGRAMS</u> are the most accurate test (95-100%) and are considered the "gold standard" when comparing all of the other diagnostic modalities. Dye is injected into the foot vein, and the venous flow is documented under fluoroscopy. Positive venograms include termination of the dye column, filling defects, excessive collaterals, or absence of part or all of the suspicious venous system.

3. <u>IMPEDANCE</u> <u>PLETHYSMOGRAPHY</u> (IPG) works by measuring <u>maximal</u> <u>venous</u> <u>output</u> <u>(MVO)</u> and <u>venous</u> <u>capacitance</u> (Fig. 4.2). The venous capacitance is calculated from the change in calf circumference as recorded by a strain gauge around the calf after a blood pressure cuff is inflated to 50 mm Hg above the knee. A patient with DVT will have a lower venous capacitance because the leg is already swollen, and subsequently there is a smaller change in volume when the cuff is inflated.

The MVO is calculated from the slope of the curve generated after the cuff is deflated. A patient with DVT will have a flatter slope, as the outflow will be slower when the cuff is deflated.

IPG is 85-95% accurate when compared to venography and is more objective than the Doppler, but it is not portable.

4. <u>DUPLEX</u> <u>SONOGRAPHY</u> has become an excellent non-invasive test for the diagnosis of deep venous thrombosis. Duplex

sonography is a combination of both Doppler flow through the venous system of the lower extremity and direct ultrasound imaging of the clot. Duplex imaging is most advantageous for proximal thrombosis above the knee and including the femoral vein. It is unreliable for the clots below the knee. The examination is examiner dependent; however, with experience duplex scanning of the venous system has become an excellent tool for ruling out significant deep venous thrombosis.

5. ^{125}I-LABELED FIBRINOGEN is best for documenting small thrombi in the soleal veins but otherwise has limited usefulness in the clinical situation because of the high degree of false negative results. Such factors as recent surgical wounds, cellulitis, hematoma, and infection interfere with the interpretation of the scan.

The scan is performed by injecting labeled human fibrinogen and scanning the legs for uptake. A positive scan is an uptake of greater than 20% as compared with the opposite leg.

Treatment

Patients with DVT should be immediately anticoagulated unless there is a major contraindication to anticoagulation. Anticoagulation is best achieved by continuous I.V. infusion of heparin. The patient should first have a loading dose that will immediately stop any further propagation of clot or possible PE. This can usually be achieved with a loading dose of 10,000 units followed by a constant infusion of 25 mg/kg/hour. The PTT is then carefully followed and the

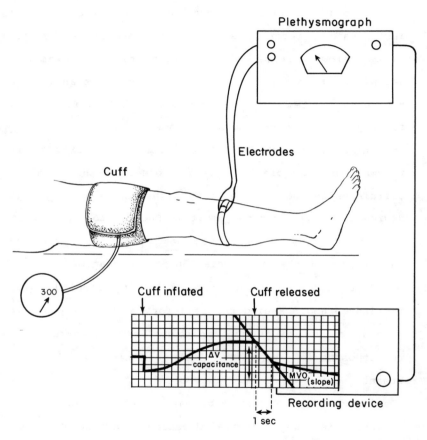

Figure 4.2.   Impedance plethysmography for determining deep venous thrombosis by measuring maximal venous output (MVO) and venous capacitance (see the text).

patient titrated to a PTT of 1.5-2 times normal (usually PTT of 80-100 seconds).

At 1 week to 10 days after anticoagulation the patient is started on oral anticoagulants (Coumadin) to maintain the PT at 1.5-2 times normal. The patient should be maintained on oral anticoagulants for at least 3 months as an outpatient.

Patients with phlegmasia cerulea (alba) dolens should have a trial of thrombolytic therapy with either streptokinase or urokinase in an effort to dissolve the clot. If this is unsuccessful, then an attempt at an ileofemoral venous thrombectomy should be made.

PULMONARY EMBOLISM

Of those patients with documented DVT, 5% will go on to have a pulmonary embolus despite adequate therapy, with a mortality of 6%. Patients with untreated DVT will develop a PE in 25% of cases, with a mortality of 35%. Unfortunately, the majority of patients with a PE have no warning signs or symptoms despite the fact that up to 85% of emboli originate in the lower extremities.

The natural history of patients with untreated PE is a 60% recurrence rate with a 35% mortality. Among those patients with adequate therapy, 20% will have a recurrence with a mortality of 5%. Because the mortality of untreated DVT and PE is so high, it is imperative that patients be diagnosed and treated quickly and aggressively.

The signs and symptoms of PE include tachypnea, chest pain, hemoptysis, tachycardia, rales, fever, friction rub, or frank shock. Common findings on work-up are infiltrates or effusion on chest x-ray, ST-T wave changes on EKG, and blood gases with a PaO_2 of less then 80 and usually a low PCO_2 as a result of the hyperventilation. A perfusion lung scan should be obtained immediately to rule out PE. A normal or low probability scan usually will rule out a PE, but an equivocal or high probability scan is only 54-70% correct and thus requires a pulmonary angiogram for confirmation.

Treatment of pulmonary emboli is the same as for DVT; immediate heparinization and subsequent oral anticoagulation for 3-6 months. Patients with massive PE and hypotensive shock should be considered for an emergent pulmonary embolectomy.

VENA CAVAL INTERRUPTION PROCEDURES

As stated above, the mortality from either untreated DVT or PE is unacceptably high, so that a mechanical device must be placed in patients who cannot be anticoagulated, to prevent possible pulmonary emboli. The three indications for vena caval interruption include

1. Recurrent PE on adequate anticoagulation;

2. Contraindication to anticoagulation (i.e., recent neurosurgery or gastrointestinal bleeding);

3. Complication of anticoagulation (i.e., gastrointestinal bleeding while on heparin).

Another relative indication for vena caval interruption involves the high-risk patient undergoing another operative procedure who has a significant history of deep venous thrombosis or pulmonary embolism. He would be considered a candidate for an interruption procedure at the same time as his other operative procedure. Because of the safety and efficacy of the Greenfield Filter, the indications for its placement have liberalized over the last several years. They include

(1) Patients with a free-floating thrombus in the inferior vena cava who are at an extraordinarily high risk for developing pulmonary embolism,

(2) Patients with metastatic carcinoma who are at significant risk of bleeding from standard anticoagulation or known to be relatively anticoagulation resistent, and finally

(3) There is some suggestion that the primary treatment of deep venous thrombosis may be a Greenfield Filter as opposed to any anticoagulation, as the long-term results of anticoagulation for the resolution of the symptoms of deep venous thrombosis are poor.

Currently the most widely used interruption device is the Greenfield Filter. The filter is a metal cage that is placed within the inferior vena cava under local anesthesia via the jugular or femoral vein with the use of fluoroscopy. With the new design of the filter, it can be placed percutaneously through a 12 French sheath. The filter is usually placed below the renal veins at the   L-3-L-4 vertebral level. The filter has a very high inferior vena caval patency rate of 95% and a low recurrent embolus rate of 2.6%.

The two commonly used external caval clips are the _Moretz clip_ (Fig. 4.3) and the Adams-Deweese clip (Fig. 4.3). Both of these clips work on the same principle of partial caval occlusion to prevent massive pulmonary embolism. They are easily applied around the cava below the renal veins at the time of abdominal exploration for other pathology. The patency rates are very high, and postoperative leg edema occurs in only 5% of cases.

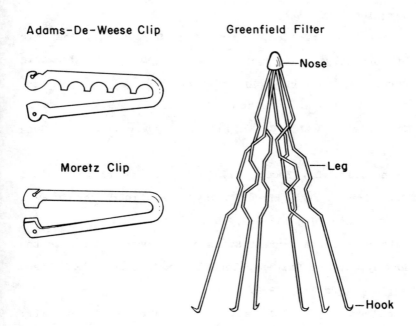

Figure 4.3.   Vena caval interruption devices.

SUGGESTED READINGS

1. Cline, W., Spradlin, S., Perry, M.: Considerations in Diagnosing Deep Venous Thrombosis. Infections in Surgery, p. 96, Aug. 1983.

2. Coon, W.: Epidemiology of Venous Thromboembolism. Ann Surg 186:149, 1977.

3. Elliot, M., Immelman, E., Benatar, S., et al.: The Role of Thrombolytic Therapy in the Management of Phlegmasia Cerulea Dolens. Br J Surg 66:422, 1979.

4. Greenfield, L., Peyton, R., Crute, S., et al.: Greenfield Vena Caval Filter Experience. Arch Surg 116:1451, 1981.

5. Greenfield, L., Zocco, J., Wilk, J., et al.: Clinical Experience with the Kim-Ray Greenfield Vena Caval Filter. Ann Surg 185:692, 1977.

6. Kakkar, V.: The Current Staus of Low Dose Heparin in the Prophylaxis of Thrombophlebitis and Pulmonary Embolism. World J Surg 2:3, 1978.

7. Nicolaides, A., Miles, C., Hoare, M., et al.: Intermittent Sequential Pneumatic Compression of the Legs and Thromboembolism Deterrent Stockings in the Prevention of Postoperative Deep Venous Thrombosis. Surgery 94:21, 1983.

8. Rosenow, E., Osmundson, P., Brown, M.: Pulmonary Embolism. Mayo Clin Proc 56:161, 1981.

9. Rosenthal, D., Cossman, D., Matsumoto, G., et al.: Prophylactic Interruption of the Inferior Vena Cava. Am J Surg 137:389, 1979.

10. Russell, J.: Prophylaxis of Postoperative Deep Vein Thrombosis and Pulmonary Embolism. _Surg Gynecol Obstet_ 157:89, 1983.

11. Sabiston, D.: Pathophysiology, Diagnosis, and Management of Pulmonary Embolism. _Am J Surg_ 138:384, 1979.

12. Salzman, E., Davies, G.: Prophylaxis of Venous Thromboembolism. _Ann Surg_ 191:207, 1980.

Chapter 5

Venous Stasis Disease and Varicose Veins

Unfortunately, patients with venous stasis ulcers usually get the lowest priority of care in surgical clinics and usually have their care delegated to the most junior member of the surgical team. As a result, their care usually ends up being suboptimal only because of the poor understanding of the pathophysiology of the disease. Venous stasis disease and varicose veins are two different disease entities, usually unrelated and requiring different therapy. The majority of these patients can be helped a great deal with the appropriate treatment.

VENOUS ANATOMY OF THE LOWER EXTREMITY

An understanding of the venous anatomy of the leg is absolutely essential to the understanding of these two diseases. The lower leg has two venous systems:

1. THE DEEP SYSTEM: The posterior tibial and peroneal veins of the lower leg drain the majority of the muscle mass of the lower leg and subsequently empty into the popliteal vein. The posterior tibial vein receives two very important perforating veins that directly drain the skin and subcutaneous tissue of the medial malleolus.

2. THE <u>SUPERFICIAL</u> <u>SYSTEM</u> (Fig. 5.1) includes the <u>greater</u> and <u>lesser</u> <u>saphenous</u> veins. The greater saphenous vein runs on the medial side of the lower leg, receives branches from the foot and at the level of the knee, and empties into the femoral vein at the fossa ovalis in the upper leg. One very important branch is a <u>posterior communicating branch</u> which communicates with the third perforator of the deep system. This branch is an important connection between the deep and superficial system in the etiology of varicose veins of the lower leg. The lesser saphenous runs posteriolateral in the lower leg and receives a lateral perforating branch before emptying into the popliteal vein.

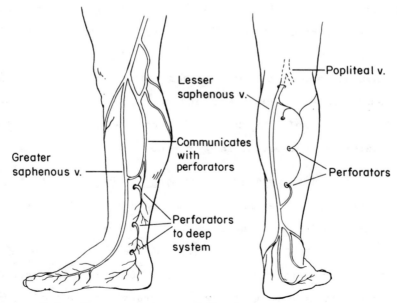

Figure 5.1   Venous anatomy of the leg.

VENOUS STASIS DISEASE

As discussed above, the primary drainage of the lower leg is via the deep venous system. Patients with venous stasis ulcers have long-standing incompetence of the perforating draining veins of the lower leg. As a result, blood flow from the deep system backs up into the skin and subcutaneous tissue of the lower leg, causing edema of the lower leg. In time, the skin breaks down and an ulcer develops (Fig. 5.2). If left untreated the ulcer will then become superficially infected. Commonly the ulcers develop near the medial malleolus where the incompetent perforators are located. Hemosiderin from the stagnant blood turns the area a dark brownish-black color. Since the superficial venous system has little to do with the drainage of this area, incompetence of the saphenous vein (varicose veins) is usually unrelated.

A small subset of patients has venous stasis disease as a result of DVT. Thrombosis and phlebitis within the deep system can result in destruction of the normal valvular mechanism and subsequent incompetence.

TREATMENT OF VENOUS STASIS DISEASE

Based upon the pathophysiology of the disease the treatment varies with the stage of the ulcer:

1. INFECTED ULCERS usually have not been treated or have been treated improperly. The patient needs to be at strict bed rest with the foot of the bed elevated for maximal lower extremity drainage. It is essential to get the edema to

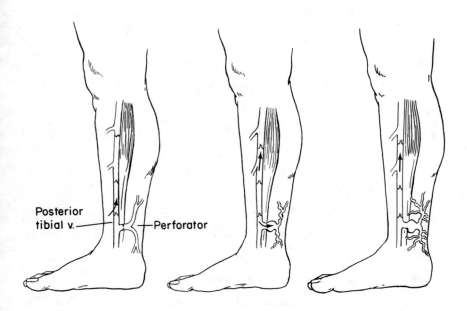

Figure 5.2.   The pathophysiology for the development of venous stasis ulcers. Incompetence of the perforating veins results in blood backup into the skin, edema of the subcutaneous tissue, skin breakdown, and subsequent ulceration.

resolve to promote tissue healing. Wet to dry saline dressings, changed four times a day, are used to debride the ulcer in addition to scrubbing the ulcer four times a day with soap and water. Usually the infection is very superficial and will respond to mechanical efforts. Antibiotics are usually unnecessary unless there is a significant component of surrounding soft tissue erythema and cellulitis. If cellulitis is present, then a broad spectrum antibiotic should be used for 5-7 days.

2. <u>CLEAN</u> <u>ULCERS</u> or those minimally infected can be treated on an outpatient basis. It is important for the patient to walk or exercise, but standing idle increases edema formation. When off their feet, patients should keep their legs elevated. A medicated compression boot commonly known as an "<u>UNNA</u> <u>BOOT</u>" (Graham-Field Surgical Co., Inc., New Hyde Park, N.Y.) is applied to the lower leg and kept in place at all times. This acts to keep compression on the lower extremity so that tissue edema does not occur. The bandage that forms the boot is medicated with zinc oxide glycerine which acts to prevent further skin breakdown and as a topical antibiotic. The boot can be left in place for up to 2 weeks and then changed. With elevation and an Unna boot, almost 100% of ulcers will eventually close. Depending on the size of the ulcer, it may take several months to heal a large ulcer.

3. THE <u>HEALED</u> <u>ULCER</u> must be treated throughout life, or it will recurr. The mainstay of treatment after the ulcer has closed is compression stockings that are individually fitted for each patient. The stockings are custom fitted to apply a venous pressure gradient which is greatest at the ankle. Since the underlying pathology (incompetent perforators) has not been corrected, the patient needs to wear the stockings at all times when erect.

4. <u>SURGICAL</u> <u>THERAPY</u> usually involves a procedure that ligates the incompetent perforators. The <u>Cockett</u> <u>procedure</u> involves a medial incision beginning behind the medial malleolus and <u>ligation</u> of the <u>incompetent</u> <u>perforators</u> as they enter the deep investing fascia of the lower leg. The procedure should be limited to younger patients in whom the ankle tissues have not yet become a chronic mass of indurated fibrous tissue. The ideal time to operate is after the ulcer has been closed with conservative therapy. The <u>Linton</u> <u>procedure</u> is based upon the same principle but requires a much more extensive dissection and subfascial ligation of the perforators. After either procedure the patient is encouraged to continue to wear custom-fitted venous pressure gradient stockings to help prevent edema in the lower leg.

Major valvular incompetence of the popliteal or femoral veins resulting in venous stasis disease is now a correctable entity due to recent advances in venous valve surgery. Either vein valve transplant from the brachial vein to the area of incompetence or valvuloplasty of the defective valve can now be performed.

VARICOSE VEINS

Varicose veins are categorized as either primary or secondary based upon the etiology of their origin.

1. PRIMARY VARICOSITIES are usually congenital, have a strong familial pattern, and are more commonly found in women. The primary defect is absence or incompetence of the saphenofemoral valve and the other valves in the greater and lesser saphenous system. In addition, the veins have a thinner, more elastic wall.

2. SECONDARY VARICOSITIES occur as a result of previous trauma or phlebitis of the deep or superficial systems that has damaged the valvular system.

The result of either primary or secondary incompetent valves is reversal of flow within the saphenous systems. Blood from the deep system is emptied into the greater saphenous vein at the saphenofemoral junction because of the incompetent saphenofemoral valve. Blood is then drained from the superficial system dependently or via the communicating veins back into the deep system. Part of this blood volume is once again drained back into the superficial system at the saphenofemoral junction, resulting in a circular motion of part of the blood volume. The end result of this circular flow pattern is chronically dilated, tortuous varicosities. Standing or sitting for prolonged periods of time or obesity aggravates the condition.

THE PATIENT WITH VARICOSE VEINS

Patients with varicose veins complain of

1. <u>Tiredness</u> or <u>heaviness</u> of the legs, especially when standing;

2. Displeasure at the <u>cosmetic</u> appearance of their legs;

3. <u>Bleeding</u> from a varicosity that has been traumatized.

A Trendelenburg test should be done to document incompetency of either the saphenofemoral valve, the valves of the perforating veins, or both (Fig. 5.3). Varicosities of the calf region are a result of incompetence within the lesser saphenous system.

TRENDELENBURG TEST

1. With the patient supine, the leg is elevated to drain the blood. A tourniquet is then applied to the upper thigh.

2. The results of the test are based upon a biphasic response after the patient stands. The first response refers to the competency of the perforating vein valves of the lower leg. The second response refers to the competency of the saphenofemoral valve after the tourniquet is removed.

   A-<u>Negative-Negative</u>. A normal response, the saphenofemoral valve is intact and the perforating vein valves are intact.

   B-<u>Negative-Positive</u>. No retrograde filling from perforators but an incompetent saphenofemoral valve.

   C-<u>Positive-Negative</u>. Incompetent perforators with a competent saphenofemoral valve.

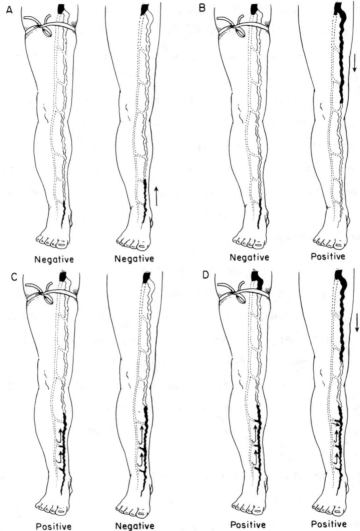

Figure 5.3. The <u>Trendelenburg</u> <u>test</u> for venous insufficiency examines for incompetency of either the saphenofemoral valve, the valves of the perforating veins or both.

D-<u>Positive-Positive</u>. Incompetency of both the perforators and the saphenofemoral valve.

(From: Schwartz, S.I., <u>Principles</u> <u>of</u> <u>Surgery</u>, ed 4, figure 22-14, pp 992-993. McGraw-Hill, New York, 1984.)

The possible treatments of varicose veins include

1. <u>CUSTOM-FITTED</u> <u>STOCKINGS</u> which apply a gradient of pressure from the ankle upward and will help for symptomatic relief of heaviness or tiredness in patients not considered candidates for surgery or sclerotherapy.

2. <u>SAPHENOUS</u> <u>VEIN</u> <u>STRIPPING</u> <u>OR</u> <u>EXCISION</u> is the mainstay of surgical therapy and corrects the underlying pathology. Surgery should only be offered to those patients considered excellent operative risks, since the majority of patients have minimal disability or are interested in cosmetic results only.

   Complete removal of the greater saphenous vein is not required, and local excision of the varicosities is an excellent alternative to complete stripping of the saphenous vein. Local excision of the varicosities preserves the main-trunk of the saphenous vein. It then can be used later if necessary as a vein graft for subsequent procedures. Complete removal of the greater saphenous vein and ligation and division of its <u>five</u> <u>major</u> <u>proximal</u> <u>tributaries</u> (Fig. 5.4) may be necessary in many patients who have extensive varicosities throughout the entire system. Major communicating veins between the deep and superficial system should also be ligated. Regardless of the method, the veins and perforating communicators should be marked by the operating surgeon prior to the surgery, with the patient in an upright position. Postoperatively the patient is kept at bed rest with the leg elevated for 24 hours. The dressings are not changed until the second postoperative day, after which a clean Ace bandage is applied and the patient is able to ambulate.

3. SCLEROTHERAPY can be used to control small varicose veins but is unreliable in major saphenous vein incompetence. The procedure involves the injection of 0.5 ml of either 3% sodium tetradecyl sulfate or sodium morrhuate into an isolated varix. The sclerosing agent is injected directly into the varix, and then a compression dressing is applied. Multiple injections can be done at one time, after which the leg is wrapped with Ace bandages. The dressings are taken down at 1 week, and residual varices are reinjected. Sclerosing should only be done by surgeons who do it frequently and are very familiar with the procedure, as it requires a commitment to rigorous follow-up and reinjections for satisfactory results.

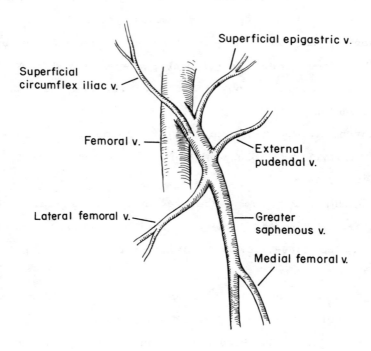

Figure 5.4. The greater saphenous vein and its proximal branches.

SUGGESTED READINGS

1. Cockett, F.B.: The Pathology and Treatment of Venous Ulcers of the Leg. Br J Surg 43:260, 1955.

2. Hobbs, J.T.: Surgery and Sclerotherapy in the Treatment of Varicose Veins. Arch Surg 109:793, 1974.

3. Hobbs, J.T.: The Treatment of Varicose Veins by Sclerosing Therapy. In Vascular Surgery, edited by R.B. Rutherford, ed 1, pp 1153-1167. W.B. Saunders Co., Philadelphia, 1977.

4. Linton, R.: Post-thrombotic Ulceration of the Lower Extremity, Its Etiology and Surgical Treatment. Ann Surg 138:415, 1953.

5. Lofgren, E.P.: The Operative Treatment of Varicose Veins. In Vascular Surgery, edited by R.B. Rutherford, ed 1, pp 1169-1175. W.B. Saunders Co., Philadelphia, 1977.

6. Raju, S.: Venous Insufficiency of the Lower Limb and Stasis Ulceration. Ann Surg 197:688, 1983.

7. Sumner, D.S.: The Hemodynamics and Pathophysiology of Venous Disease. In Vascular Surgery, edited by R.B. Rutherford, ed 1, pp 157-159. W.B. Saunders Co., Philadelphia, 1977.

8. Taheri, S., Elias, S.: Vein Valve Transplant. Contemp Surg 22:17, 1983.

Chapter 6

Acute Arterial Insufficiency: Embolus Versus Thrombosis

The early diagnosis and aggressive early treatment of patients with acute arterial insufficiency is especially important because the final outcome is dependent on the duration of tissue ischemia. The differentiation between embolus and thrombosis is important, since treatment is different for the two types of lesions. Duration of ischemia as related to outcome in one large series of patients with emboli revealed the following:

Diagnosis and embolectomy:

Within 8 hours of occurrence---20% ischemic complications;

8-24 hours after occurrence----32% ischemic complications;

1-7 days after occurrence------43% ischemic complications.

HISTORY

The <u>most</u> <u>common</u> <u>cause</u> of acute arterial insufficiency is an <u>embolus</u> <u>from</u> <u>the</u> <u>heart</u>. Cardiac sources include clot that forms as a result of arrhythmias (usually atrial fibrillation), mitral stenosis, or mural thrombus from a fresh myocardial infarction. Rarely, plaque from an arterial aneurysm will embolize.

Emboli to the lower extremity are 10 times more common than those to the upper extremity, with the <u>most</u> <u>common</u> <u>site</u> being the <u>superficial</u> <u>femoral</u> <u>arteries</u>.

The history of the event will help to establish whether the cause is embolus or thrombosis. Important historical facts include

1. The <u>time</u> <u>of</u> <u>onset</u> of <u>pain</u>, loss of sensation, or change in temperature. Many patients will give the exact time of onset because of the sudden nature of the acute onset of pain.

2. As discussed above, it is important to establish a past history of <u>heart</u> <u>disease</u> including arrhythmias or MI.

3. A <u>previous</u> <u>history</u> of <u>peripheral</u> <u>vascular</u> <u>disease</u>, especially a past history of claudication in the affected extremity. Patients with this type of history most likely have had a thrombosis of an already compromised vessel.

4. A recent <u>episode</u> <u>of</u> <u>hypotension</u> or dehydration usually favors thrombosis of a compromised vessel.

<u>PHYSICAL</u> <u>EXAMINATION</u>

Arterial emboli commonly <u>lodge</u> <u>at</u> <u>arterial</u> <u>bifurcations</u> of the major vessels including femoral, iliac, aorta, popliteal, and less commonly brachial, renal, mesenteric, and carotid. Ischemic findings occur to the area distal to the obstruction. The physical findings are classically described by the five P's:

1. <u>PAIN</u> is constant and is associated with any movement of the extremity.

2. PALLOR: A pale, yellowish tone to the extremity below the site of obstruction.

3. PULSELESS below the site of occlusion or as compared with the opposite extremity in conjunction with poor capillary filling.

4. PARESTHESIAS: Anoxia to the peripheral nerves resulting in paresthesias is an early and sensitive sign of inadequate arterial blood supply.

5. PARALYSIS is a very late and grave sign. A majority of patients presenting with paralysis have necrotic muscle and will never regain function or will require an amputation.

The other important local findings include a cold extremity below the site of obstruction as compared with proximal areas and with the other side. Collapsed superficial veins are further evidence for poor arterial inflow. Evidence of heart disease, irregular rhythm, and chronic vascular insufficiency should be closely evaluated.

DIAGNOSIS AND TREATMENT

Laboratory values are of little benefit except where severe muscle necrosis has occurred resulting in elevated creatinine phosphatase. All patients should have chest x-rays and cardiograms to help evaluate the cardiac status.

If the diagnosis of acute arterial insufficiency is suspected:

1. The patient should be immediately heparinized (while in the emergency room if necessary) until further diagnostic

testing or treatment has been decided. An intravenous bolus of 10,000 units and continuous drip of 1000 units/hour of heparin will <u>prevent</u> <u>subsequent</u> <u>propagation</u> <u>of</u> <u>clot</u> both distally and proximal to the occlusion. Propagation of clot can cause local collateral vessels to thrombose and cause additional ischemia.

2. An <u>arteriogram</u> should be done if there is any question that the cause may be a thrombosis and not an embolus. When a compromised vessel has thrombosed, the surgical procedure to correct the occlusion becomes much more complex and usually involves bypass grafting. <u>Thrombectomy</u> alone is not sufficient without correcting the underlying cause. In this setting, knowledge of the peripheral anatomy is critical prior to surgery.

3. In those patients with an obvious embolus, an emergent <u>embolectomy</u> should be done under local anesthesia. As discussed above, duration of ischemia can be the critical element in the final outcome. In most series, an embolectomy done under local anesthesia has an in hospital mortality of 20-30%. Mortality is so high because of the severity of the coexisting cardiac disease in association with the release of toxic metabolites when flow is reestablished. Known as the "<u>reperfusion</u> <u>phenomenon</u>," local metabolites and by-products of ischemic muscle, including potassium, lactic acid, lysozymes, and creatinine phosphatase, are released into

the circulation with reperfusion and can have severe systemic effects. Because of this phenomenon many surgeons will catheterize the femoral vein at the time of a groin embolectomy and discard the first 200-300 ml of venous blood.

4. When severe ischemia is present for an extended period of time, cell membrane damage occurs with leakage of fluid into the interstitium. The resulting edema can cause a "<u>compartment</u> <u>syndrome</u>" whereby tissues cannot swell within closed fascial compartments and further necrosis occurs. Pressures within the lower extremity compartments can become very high, resulting in severe muscle necrosis and tissue loss. Faciotomies that relieve the high pressure and allow the edematous tissue to expand should always be considered at the time of surgery.

Because of the severity of the associated cardiac disease, the <u>mortality</u> of acute lower extremity ischemia is 20-30%. As a result of this high mortality, other therapeutic options are now being investigated for acute arterial insufficiency. The first of these is a regimen of high dose heparin initially, followed by elective surgery 1 week later, as descibed by Blaisdell et al. In this series the limb survival rate was the same as with embolectomy, but the mortality was much lower.

The other therapeutic option, now being used by many centers, is pharmacological lysis of the clot with <u>intra-arterial</u> <u>infusion</u> of <u>streptokinase</u> or <u>urokinase</u>. This treatment is particularly attractive in patients with grafts that have clotted or thrombosis of a compromised vessel. It allows time for improving the patient's condition, establishing the underlying cause for the thrombosis, and obtaining the necessary preoperative studies. Surgery is then done electively to correct the underlying defect.

NATURAL HISTORY AND LONG TERM THERAPY

Those patients with an embolus of cardiac origin should be maintained on chronic anticoagulation. The 5-year recurrence rate is 20% in patients anticoagulated as opposed to 40% in patients not anticoagulated. In those patients with a thrombosis or no obvious source for an embolus, evidence is lacking to support chronic anticoagulation.

Unfortunately, because of the associated cardiac disease, the long-term outlook for the majority of these patients is poor. The average survival for patients with an embolus is 3.1 years as compared with 17 years for an age matched population with no history of an embolus.

SUGGESTED READINGS

1. Berni, G., Bandyk, D., Zierler, E., et al.: Strepto-kinase Treatment of Acute Arterial Occlusion. Ann Surg 192:185, 1983.

2. Blaisdell, F., Steele, M., Allen, R.: Management of Acute Lower Extremity Arterial Ischemia Due to Embolism and Thrombosis. Surgery 84:822, 1978.

3. Cambria, R., Abbott, W.: Acute Arterial Thrombosis of the Lower Extremity. Arch Surg 119:784 1984.

4. Dale, A.: Differential Management of Acute Peripheral Arterial Ischemia. J Vasc Surg 1:269, 1984.

5. Elliot, J., Hageman, J., Szilagyi, D., et al.: Arterial Embolization: Problems of Source, Multiplicity, Recurrence, and Delayed Treatment. Surgery 88:883, 1980.

6. Jarrett, F., Dacumas, G., Crummy, A., et al.: Late Appearance of Arterial Emboli: Diagnosis and Management. Surgery 86:898, 1979.

7. McPhail, N., Fratesi, S., Barber, G., et al.: Management of Acute Thromboembolic Limb Ischemia. Surgery 93:381, 1983.

8. Rush, D., Gewertz, B., Chien-Tai Lu, et al.: Selective Infusion of Streptokinase for Arterial Thrombosis. Surgery 93:828, 1983.

9. Silvers, L., Royster, T., Mulcare, R.: Peripheral Arterial Emboli and Factors in Their Recurrence Rate. Ann Surg 192:232, 1980.

10. Wolfson, R., Kumpe, D., Rutherford, R.: Role of Intra-arterial Streptokinase in the Treatment of Arterial Thromboembolism. Arch Surg 119:697, 1984.

Chapter 7

Vascular Trauma

Vascular injuries like other trauma occur as a result of either gunshot wounds, sharp-edged instruments, or blunt trauma. In multiple reports on the etiology for arterial injuries, gunshot wounds are the most common cause of artery injury.

The most common site of injury is the extremities, followed by the neck, aorta, and visceral vessels, respectively. Associated injuries such as neurological injuries, chest injuries, and intraabdominal injuries are the major determinants of the survival. Major arterial injuries are frequently associated with other injuries as follows: significant venous injuries, 34%; major nerve injury, 18%; separate arteries, 7%; lung and abdominal viscera, 39%; and shock, 36%.

The types of vascular injury vary from complete transection to partial laceration, contusion, or spasm. Vascular injuries are also frequently associated with major long bone injuries. Acute arterial insufficiency is a very morbid condition and has major local and systemic manifestations (Chapter 6). For this reason, identification and treatment of vascular injuries is critical to long-term morbidity and mortality.

Signs and symptoms suggesting arterial injury include

1. Diminished or absent distal pulses;

2. History of persistent arterial bleeding;

3. Large or expanding hematoma;

4. Major hemorrhage with hypotension or shock;

5. Bruit at or distal to the suspected site of injury;

6. Injury of anatomical related nerve;

7. Anatomical proximity of the wound to a major blood vessel.

Unfortunately, the presence of pulses does not rule out proximal arterial injury, as up to 15% of patients with proven arterial injuries have normal distal pulses and pressures.

After resuscitation of the patient, preoperative or intraoperative arteriography is extremely helpful in identifying the exact location and nature of the arterial injury. In unstable patients where time for angiography is not possible, immediate surgery is indicated to identify the source and the nature of the arterial injury, with intraoperative angiography as a valuable adjunct.

GENERAL PRINCIPLES

When operating on patients with vascular injury, several basic principles should be adhered to:

1. Proximal and distal control of the injured blood vessel is essential prior to exploration of the hematoma or bleeding area to prevent ongoing and subsequent blood losses.

2. With any significant arterial injury, resection and debridement of the artery and end-to-end anastomosis is usually preferable when more than 50% of the vessel is damaged.

3. Most vessels can be mobilized several centimeters, thereby obviating the need for a graft. If a graft is required, <u>autogenous tissue is usually preferable</u> depending on the site of the injury. Synthetic grafts are contraindicated in the setting of intraabdominal bowel contamination.

4. One must make sure that distal clots are removed. A <u>completion arteriogram</u> is helpful in most cases to document distal flow.

5. Concomitant venous injuries should usually be repaired if accessible.

6. The lack of distal pulses or a cool extremity should <u>never be blamed on spasm</u> without appropriate documentation (arteriogram) to prove that no intrinsic lesion remains.

<u>SPECIFIC ARTERIAL INJURIES</u>

<u>Carotid Artery Trauma</u>

The most important factor in the management of patients with carotid artery injury is the preoperative neurological status of the patient. Patients have been grouped into three categories:

1. Those with carotid injuries and no neurological deficit;

2. Those with a mild neurological deficit;

3. Those with a severe neurological deficit.

In those patients with no neurological deficit or mild deficit, repair of the carotid artery is usually safe and is recommended.   In those with a severe neurological deficit, particularly in those with altered consciousness, there is a significant risk of converting a bland cerebral infarct into a hemorrhagic infarct if blood flow is restored.   Therefore, under these circumstances ligation of the carotid is usually recommended instead of repair.

The most important part of the preoperative workup in patients with carotid artery injuries is the decision to do a preoperative angiogram if time permits.   The neck is divided into three zones when making these therapeutic decisions:

1. Zone I at the base of the neck;

2. Zone II base of neck to angle of mandible;

3. Zone III in the upper portion of the neck above the mandible.

In patients with zone I and III injuries, preoperative arteriography is usually recommended to document any injuries at the thoracic outlet or high in the neck. Patients with zone II injuries usually can undergo exploration and on-table angiography if necessary.

Blunt injuries to the carotid can occur in association with hyperextension injuries of the neck, which can produce extensive stretching, contusion, and subsequent thrombosis of the internal carotid artery.   These types of injuries can be insidious in onset and may not occur until several hours after the initial injury. Signs and symptoms associated with blunt trauma of the carotid include

1. Hematoma of the neck;

2. Horner's syndrome;

3. Lucid interval after injury, followed by unconsciousness;

4. Transient ischemic event;

5. Limb paralysis or paresis in the alert patient.

Preoperative diagnostic arteriography is critical to excluding these types of injuries.

INTRAABDOMINAL INJURIES

Injuries to the aorta and its major branches can be extremely difficult to handle. An aortic injury can occasionally be repaired by patch graft angioplasty or end-to-end anastomosis, but in most cases it requires a synthetic graft because of the inability to mobilize the aorta and the inability to obtain autogenous tissue of the correct size match. Iliac arteries are somewhat more mobile and frequently can be repaired by end-to-end anastomosis, depending on the amount of tissue loss. One of the major problems associated with aortic and iliac injuries is the association with bowel injuries and its concomitant bacterial contamination. In this setting, the placement of an intraabdominal synthetic graft is contraindicated, so that other extra-anatomical routes for revascularization of the lower extremities is indicated; i.e., an iliac artery injury that would otherwise require a graft should be oversewn and a femoro-femoral or axillo-femoral graft placed to restore blood to the lower extremity.

Injuries to the renal arteries, superior mesenteric artery, or celiac axis can usually be repaired with the use of an autogenous graft if necessary. All attempts should be made to preserve renal blood supply. A nephrectomy should not be performed without documentation of a contralateral kidney.

Venous injuries are repaired when possible with lateral venography. Inferior vena caval injuries are best controlled with a side-biting (Satinsky) clamp and repaired primarily. Inferior vena cava ligation can be performed but is usually poorly tolerated. Common iliac vein injuries should be repaired if possible.

Retroperitoneal hematomas in association with blunt trauma (pelvic fractures) should usually not be disturbed. Arteriography and embolization of the feeding vessels is a better therapeutic option than operative exploration of pelvic hematomas that result from blunt trauma.

Extremity Vascular Injuries

Injuries to the subclavian axillary, brachial artery, femoral artery, superficial femoral artery, profundus femoral, and popliteal arteries should always be repaired if possible. Injuries to the radial or ulnar arteries should be repaired if the other vessel is not functioning or is also injured. Injuries to an isolated tibial vessel can usually be ligated or repaired if other tibial vessels are also injured. However, in the majority of cases isolated tibial vessels can be ligated.

Injuries to the popliteal artery are particularly morbid as the amputation rate approaches 50% with ligation or failure to repair the artery. Injury to the popliteal vein should also be repaired as the association with venous gangrene, severe leg swelling, and compromise of the arterial repair is significant.

Preoperative arteriography is extremely helpful with all of these types of injuries, and completion arteriography is essential for documentation of good distal flow. As mentioned earlier, the presence of distal pulses does not rule out proximal arterial injury, and the absence of peripheral pulses after arterial repair mandates a completion arteriogram before the patient leaves the operating room.

Grafts of choice in the extremities are usually autogenous tissue, which in most cases is the saphenous vein. In patients with venous injuries to the lower extremities, the contralateral saphenous vein is used as the graft. The ipsilateral saphenous vein is not used, as it may become the major venous outflow tract if the venous repair fails or if the venous injury requires ligation.

Patients with combined arterial and venous injuries should have a four-compartment fasciotomy, as the development of a compartment syndrome with combined injuries is extremely high.

SUGGESTED READINGS

1. Perry, M.O., Thal, E.R., Shires, G.T.:   Management of Arterial Injuries. Ann Surg 173:403-408, 1971.

2. Rich, N.M., Baugh, J.H., Hughes, C.W.:   Acute Arterial Injuries in Vietnam: 1,000 cases. J Trauma 10:359-369, 1970.

3. Hughes, C.W., Baugh, J.H.: Management of Venous Injuries. Ann Surg 171:724-730, 1970.

4. Thal, E.R., Snyder, W.H., Hays, R.J., Perry, M.O.: Management of Carotid Artery Injuries.   Surgery 76:955-962, 1974.

5. Bongard, F., Dubrow, T., Klein, S.:   Vascular Injuries in the Urban Battleground: Experience at a Metropolitan Trauma Center. Ann Vasc Surg 4(5):415-418, 1990.

6. Louridas, G., Perry, M.O.:   Basic Data Related to Vascular Trauma. Ann Vasc Surg 3(4):397-399, 1989.

7. Mattox, K.L., Feliciano, D.V., Burch, J., et al.:   Five Thousand Seven Hundred Sixty Cardiovascular Injuries in 4459 Patients.   Epidemologic Evolution 1958 to 1987. Ann Surg 209(6):698-707, 1989.

Chapter 8

Cerebral Vascular Disease

Stroke is the third most common cause of death in the United States, with a rate that is increasing as the population grows older. The risk factors include hypertension, smoking, obesity, and hyperlipidemias. The prognosis for a stroke is as follows: 80% will survive the initial event of which

29% will function normally;

36% will be able to return to work;

18% will be unable to work but take care of themselves;

4% will require total custodial care.

The natural history of those patients sustaining a stroke suggests that only 50% of patients will be alive at 5 years, one-half of whom will die as result of a recurrent stroke. Of those surviving a stroke, 25% will have another stroke for which the mortality is 62%. Because the sequelae of a stroke can be so devastating, any patient with symptoms of cerebrovascular disease or any patient who has sustained a stroke should be aggressively worked up in hopes of finding a correctable lesion.

Patients with cerebrovascular disease can be classified by clinical presentation in the following manner:

1. <u>Asymptomatic</u> <u>bruits</u> over the carotid artery can be found in many patients with no clinical symptoms of extracranial cerebrovascular disease. The bruit results from a stenosis usually at the bifurcation of the common carotid artery.

2. <u>Transient</u> <u>ischemic</u> <u>attacks</u> <u>(TIAs)</u> are defined as any transient neurological deficit lasting from several seconds to many hours and may include complete hemiparesis or just a small loss of sensation to an extremity. They are quite variable, covering the entire spectrum of neurological dysfunction. By definition a TIA can <u>last</u> <u>no</u> <u>longer</u> <u>than</u> <u>24</u> <u>hours</u>, after which it is considered a stroke. <u>Amaurosis</u> <u>fugax</u> is a type of transient attack whereby the patient experiences <u>temporary</u> <u>monocular</u> <u>blindness</u> usually described as a "shade coming down over the eye." Amaurosis fugax results from the embolization of platelets or cholesterol to the ophthalmic artery (a branch off the internal carotid artery). The most common source of these emboli is an <u>ulcerated</u> <u>plaque</u> of the common carotid artery where it bifurcates into the internal and external carotid arteries. Funduscopic examinations during these episodes have documented the plaques as they traverse the retina. Originally decribed by Hollenhorst, these plaques now carry the name of <u>Hollenhorst</u> <u>bodies</u>.

3. <u>Stroke</u> <u>in</u> <u>evolution</u> is a neurological deficit that progresses or fluctuates while the patient is under observation.

4. Frank stroke (completed stroke) is a deficit that is no longer changing, which has persisted for longer than 24 hours.

PATHOPHYSIOLOGY OF STROKES AND TIAs

The two most common mechanisms causing strokes and TIAs are

1. Hypoperfusion from a tight stenosis in the common carotid artery resulting in brain ischemia in the distribution of the artery on that side.

2. Embolization of plaque or platelets off an ulcerated lesion in the carotid artery.

Other less common mechanisms include hypotension, kinking of the carotid artery, anemia, trauma, thrombocytopenia, cardiac arrhythmia, or subclavian steal.

The majority of patients have ischemic strokes (by either an embolus or low flow) as compared with a relatively small number of hemorrhagic strokes secondary to hypertension.

Lesions of the common carotid are usually localized to the common carotid and its bifurcation into the external and internal carotid arteries. The plaque usually extends up into both vessels for a short distance and ends roughly 2 cm into the internal carotid with a posterior flap. Because the lesion is so well localized, it is amenable to local resection of the plaque via an endarterectomy of that segment of artery.

TRANSIENT ISCHEMIC ATTACKS

The treatment of TIAs is based upon data about the natural history of untreated patients and the possibility of eventual stroke.

Of those patients with documented TIAs or amaurosis fugax, approximately 35% will go on to have a stroke within their lifetime. A majority of these strokes (50%) occur within 1 year of the first TIA. After the first year, the stroke risk is about 5% per year.

The results of the North American Symptomatic Carotid Endarterectomy Trial in which patients were prospectively randomized to medical therapy or surgery were as follows: 24% of patients with symptoms and high-grade carotid lesions sustained a stroke within 18 months versus 7% for surgery.

The clinical findings of TIAs and amaurosis are described above. A bruit over the carotid artery found in conjunction with a history of a TIA is very significant for a correctable carotid lesion. High-pitch bruits are more suggestive of a tight stenosis, but patients without bruits and a history of TIAs may have significant extracranial cerebrovascular disease in the form of

1. A very tight stenosis where a bruit is no longer present;
2. An ulcerated plaque that is throwing emboli without a significant stenosis;
3. An occluded carotid with distal thrombus throwing clot;
4. A more proximal lesion at the aortic arch or innominate artery;

5. Cardiac disease throwing clot, i.e., atrial fibrillation, myocardial infarction, ventricular aneurysm, arrhythmia.

All patients with a strong history of a TIA or amaurosis should undergo contrast studies by either digital subtraction intravenous methods or standard arteriography. The study should include a look at all of the carotid artery including its course through the skull, the middle cerebral arteries, and the aortic arch in search of a correctable lesion. Contrast studies are still the gold standard for determining significant disease. The role of noninvasive diagnostic studies is discussed below. Patients with a lesion should have it corrected within a short time after diagnosis.

ASYMPTOMATIC BRUITS AND ASYMPTOMATIC LESIONS

The treatment of asymptomatic high-grade carotid stenosis remains controversial. Two on-going prospective randomized studies of asymptomatic high-grade carotid lesions are currently in progress, the results of which are currently not available. The issue is whether or not the stroke rate for asymptomatic lesions is high enough to warrant surgery. Current data from prospective studies of high-grade lesions using a duplex scan suggest that 50% of patients with greater than 80% stenosis will occlude the artery within 48 months. However, at the time of the occlusion of the carotid approximately one-third to one-half of the patients will undergo a stroke. So therefore, approximately 15-20% of patients with a high-grade carotid lesions will sustain a stroke. Unfortunately there is no way of predicting which patients will sustain a stroke, so that in operating in all of the patients 4 out of 5 of the patients probably do not need the surgery. Hopefully the results of the prospective on-going studies will resolve this controversary.

CAROTID ENDARTERECTOMY (CEA)

The current <u>indications</u> for CEA include the following groups of patients found to have correctable lesions:

1. Patients with TIAs;

2. Patients undergoing coronary artery bypass grafting with bilateral high-grade carotid stenoses;

3. Some patients with asymptomatic high-grade unilateral or bilateral stenoses;

4. Stable stroke patients with an obvious lesion in the territory of the side of the stroke. Carotid endarterectomy in these patients is usually done 2-6 weeks after the acute stroke.

<u>Contraindications</u> for CEA include:

1. Acute profound stroke;

2. Stroke in evolution.

The operative mortality for CEA is about 1%, with a stroke rate of about 1-2% depending on the series reported. The operative mortality in the setting of an acute large stroke is 20-30%. The procedure involves exposing the common, internal, and external carotid arteries in the neck and endarterectomizing the plaque. Patients may require a temporary "shunt" during the operative procedure to maintain blood supply to that side of the brain while the endarterectomy is being performed. Different surgeons have different approaches to "shunting" during carotid surgery. Some surgeons shunt all patients, while others selectively shunt based upon electroencephalographic monitoring or back pressure measurements.

SUBCLAVIAN STEAL SYNDROME

This syndrome should be considered in the differential diagnosis of any patient with vertebral-basilar symptoms such as dizziness, fainting, or vertigo. Symptoms classically occur with arm exercise.

The pathophysiology of the syndrome is a manifestation of collateral blood supply to the upper extremity when the proximal subclavian artery is occluded. Blood collateralizes to the left arm by "stealing" it from the brain's posterior circulation (Fig. 8.1).

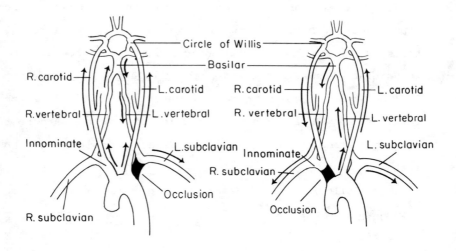

Proximal left subclavian occlusion   Innominate occlusion
     with left subclavian steal   with right subclavian steal

Figure 8.1.   The collateral pathways that result in subclavian "steal" syndrome: carotid artery----> circle of Willis----> retrograde through the basilar artery----> retrograde through the vertebral artery ----> into the subclavian artery.

The syndome occurs much more frequently on the left side but can occur on the right with an innominate artery occlusion.

NONINVASIVE CEREBROVASCULAR TESTING

Noninvasive testing of all types of arterial disease is rapidly changing as instrumentation becomes more sophisticated. Different noninvasive labs rely on different tests which are very dependent on the experience of the technician. The advent of digital intravenous arteriography (DIVA-computerized subtraction enhanced imaging) which requires only an intravenous injection of dye may make most of the current noninvasive techniques obsolete in the future.

The following is a description of some of the more common noninvasive tests used for cerebrovascular evaluation:

1. Oculoplethysmography is an indirect measurement of pulse delay within the ophthalmic artery. Since the ophthalmic artery is a branch off the internal carotid artery, delay in the pulse as compared with the ipsilateral external carotid artery or as compared with the other side would suggest a significant obstruction within the internal artery. The oculoplethysmograph works by measuring changes in the volume of the eye during arterial pulsations. The pulse in the ear is measured simultaneously as a measure of the external carotid flow. The test has a high false-negative rate and is only used in conjunction with other noninvasive testing.

2. <u>Periorbital</u> <u>blood</u> <u>flow</u> (Fig. 8.2) using a bidirectional Doppler can determine a significant stenosis within the internal carotid artery. Blood flow through the ophthalmic artery is normally toward the eye via the ophthalmic artery, but with a significant proximal stenosis, <u>flow</u> <u>is</u> <u>reversed</u> within the ophthalmic artery as a means of providing collateral circulation to the brain (Fig. 8.2).

3. <u>Duplex</u> <u>scanning</u> <u>of</u> <u>the</u> <u>carotid</u> <u>artery</u> is now considered the best of the noninvasive tests to document extracerebral vascular disease. Flow velocity is determined by waveform analysis as recorded by a continuous wave Doppler subjected to spectral analysis. In addition to the waveform analysis, a pulsed Doppler is used to determine blood velocity and volume of flow. Analysis of the waveform by a Fourier analysis is very accurate in detecting both stenosis and flow disturbances. Direct imaging of the carotid is done noninvasively with the computer-enhanced image of a high-resolution B mode scanner.

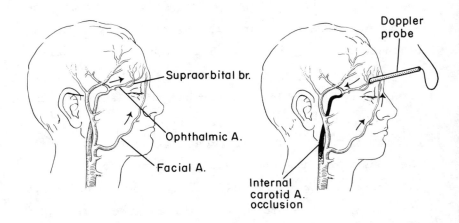

Normal direction of flow through ophthalmic artery

Reversal of flow with internal carotid artery occlusion as detected by directional Doppler

Figure 8.2. Periorbital Doppler to determine flow within the ophthalmic artery. In the presence of a significant proximal stenosis, flow is reversed as a means of providing collateral circulation to the brain. The collateral circuit includes flow from

external carotid artery ---> frontal and temporal arteries ---> supraorbital branches ---> ophthalmic artery (reversed flow) ---> distal internal carotid artery ---> brain.

SUGGESTED READINGS

1. David, N.J.:   Amaurosis Fugax and After. In <u>Neuro-</u>
    <u>Ophthalmology</u>, vol IX, chapter 2, pp 8-28. C.V. Mosby,
    St Louis, 1977.

2. DeWeese, J.A., Rob, C.G., Satran, R., et al.: Results of
    Carotid Endarterectomies for Transient Ischemic Attacks-
    Five Years Later. <u>Ann</u> <u>Surg</u> 178:258-264, 1973.

3. Hertzer,   N.R.,   Beven,   E.G.,   Benjamin,   S.P.:
    Ultramicroscopic Ulcerations and Thrombi of the Carotid
    Bifurcation. <u>Arch</u> <u>Surg</u> 112:1394-1402, 1977.

4. Hertzer,   N.R.,   Beven, E.G.,   Young, J.R.,   et al.:
    Incidental Asymptomatic Carotid Bruits in Patients
    Scheduled for Peripheral Vascular Reconstruction:
    Results of Cerebral and Coronary Angiography. <u>Surgery</u>
    96:535-544, 1984.

5. Hollenhorst,   R.W.: Significance of Bright Plaques in
    the Retinal Arterioles. <u>JAMA</u> 178:123-129, 1961.

6. Kistler,   J.P., Ropper, A.H., Heros, R.C.: Therapy of
    Ischemic   Cerebral   Vascular   Disease   Due   to
    Atherothrombosis. Part I. <u>N</u> <u>Engl</u> <u>J</u> <u>Med</u> 311:27-34, 1984.
    Part II. <u>N</u> <u>Engl</u> <u>J</u> <u>Med</u> 311:100-105, 1984.

7. Malone, J.M., Bean, B., Laguna, J., et al.: Diagnosis of
    Carotid   Artery   Stenosis.   Comparison   of
    Oculoplethysmography   and   Doppler   Supraorbital
    Examination. <u>Ann</u> <u>Surg</u> 191:347-354, 1980.

8. Matsumoto,   N., Whishant, J.P., Kurland, L.T., et al.:

Natural History of Stoke in Rochester, Minnesota 1955-1968: An Extension of a Previous Study, 1945-1954. Stroke 4:20-29, 1973.

9. Moore, W.S., Boren, C.B., Malone, J.M., et al.: Natural History of Nonstenotic Asymptomatic Ulcerative Lesions of the Carotid Artery. Arch Surg 113:1352-1359, 1978.

10. Sumner, D.S., Russell, J.B., Ramsey, D.E., et al.: Noninvasive Diagnosis of Extracranial Carotid Arterial Disease. Arch Surg 114:122-1229, 1979.

11. Thompson, J.E., Talkington, C.M.: Carotid Endarterectomy. Ann Surg 184:1-15, 1976.

12. Whittemore, A.D., Kauffman, J.L., Kohler, T.R., Mannick, J.A.: Routine EEG Monitoring during Carotid Endarterectomy. Ann Surg 197:707-713, 1983.

13. Wolf, P.A., Kannel, W.B., Sorlie, P., et al.: Asymptomatic Carotid Bruit and Risk of Stroke: The Framingham Study. JAMA 245:1442-1445, 1981.

14. Yao, J.T.: Uses of the Vascular Laboratory. Drug Ther 23-34, Jan 1982.

Chapter 9

Abdominal Aortic Aneurysms

Abdominal aortic aneurysms (AAAs) arise <u>below</u> <u>the</u> <u>renal</u> <u>arteries</u> and are due to atherosclerosis in more than 95% of cases. Why some patients develop occlusive disease as opposed to aneurysmal dilation of the aorta is still unknown. However, significant data exist suggesting that AAAs are a manifestation of a systemic disorder in elastin metabolism and probably are genetically determined. Pathology routinely reveals laminated clot and mural thrombus in the presence of a very thin aortic wall. AAAs are frequently familial, are more common in men, are coexistent with hypertension in 40% of patients, and are associated with other peripheral aneurysms in 20% of cases.

<u>NATURAL HISTORY</u>

Two series on the natural history of untreated AAAs are important to the understanding of why we treat AAAs aggressively.

1. Estes, 1950

   -The 5-, 10-, and 15-year survival of 102 untreated patients with AAAs was 9%, 0%, and 0%, respectively.

-The rupture rate was 20% within the first year and 40-50% within the first 4-5 years after diagnosis.

-As the aneurysm increases in size the rupture rate increases exponentially such that at 6 cm the rate rapidly increases.

2. Szilagyi, 1966

-In 223 untreated patients:

    < 6 cm-----19.5% rupture rate----55% mortality;

    > 6 cm-----43% rupture rate------90.1% mortality.

-Repair of the aneurysm doubled the life expectancy.

-The most common cause of death was rupture in 35% of patients, and the second most common cause was coronary artery disease in 17% of patients.

In contrast, recent results of surgical treatment in 920 patients, with an operative mortality of 1.4%, revealed 5-, 10-, and 15-year survivals of 63%, 38%, and 18%, respectively.

CLINICAL PRESENTATION

Most patients present with an asymptomatic pulsatile abdominal mass found by themselves, their primary physician, or discovered with sonogram or CT scanning done for other reasons. History is usually only important for associated cardiovascular disease. Physical exam usually reveals the AAA, which should be measured and recorded. Not infrequently a pulsatile mass in a thin female will be the aortic pulse transmitted through a normal pancreas or pancreatic mass. Do not forget to palpate for associated peripheral aneurysms, especially popliteal aneurysms.

WHAT <u>DIAGNOSTIC</u> <u>TEST</u> <u>TO</u> <u>ORDER?</u>

An accurate and easily obtainable test is the abdominal <u>sonogram</u>, which is 95% accurate to within 0.5 cm.

Other tests include

1. <u>Physical</u> <u>exam</u>, which is 85% accurate to within 1 cm, depending on the examiner and the patient's habitus.

2. <u>Cross-table</u> <u>abdominal</u> <u>lateral</u> <u>x-ray</u>, which will frequently show the calcified external aortic wall as it projects anterior to the spine.

3. <u>CT</u> <u>scan</u> with contrast, which is an excellent diagnostic test and probably most accurate in determining true diameter.

4. <u>Arteriography</u> should not be used as a diagnostic test as it usually does not visualize the aneurysm because of the intraluminal clot. When the decision has been made that the patient will require surgery, arteriography may be obtained to further define the associated vascular anatomy, i.e., the number and location of the renal arteries, renal artery involvement in the aneurysm or stenosis, patency of the inferior mesenteric artery, possible iliac aneurysms, and distal runoff below the aorta.

TREATMENT

<u>Asymptomatic</u> <u>aneurysms</u> <u>5</u> <u>cm</u> <u>or</u> <u>larger</u> <u>should</u> <u>be</u> <u>electively</u> <u>repaired</u>. While some vascular surgeons feel that any aneurysm 4 cm or larger should be repaired, patients

with small AAAs should be followed very carefully with sonograms every 3 to 6 months. Growth of 1/2 cm or greater in any six month period is an indication for repair.

Preoperative Preparation

1. AAA repair is a major operative procedure, and the patient's cardiac and pulmonary function should be maximized before surgery.

2. An <u>arterial</u> <u>catheter</u> should be placed preoperatively for intraoperative blood pressure monitoring and arterial blood gas measurements. A <u>baseline</u> <u>arterial</u> <u>blood</u> <u>gas</u> should be obtained.

3. A mechanical <u>bowel</u> <u>prep</u> is preferred by some surgeons, starting the night prior to surgery.

4. <u>Paregoric</u>, several drops in 10 ml of water, should be given the night before surgery to help keep the small bowel minimally dilated.

5. <u>Broad</u> <u>spectrum</u> <u>antibiotics</u>, usually a cephalosporin, should be given I.V. on call to the operating room.

POSTOPERATIVE CARE AND COMPLICATIONS

The patients usually spend days in an intensive care unit with careful monitoring of the peripheral pulses. The nasogastric tube is removed after the ileus has resolved. Rare but morbid complications that should be specifically watched for include:

1. <u>Renal</u> <u>insufficiency</u> can be from hypovolemia, but renal artery occlusion or embolization as a result of aortic

cross-clamping must be considered.

2. Ischemic colitis is a result of inadequate blood flow to the colon when the inferior mesenteric artery has been ligated without enough collateral flow.   Most patients tolerate IMA ligation unless they have had a previous colon resection.   Ischemic colitis usually presents as early persistent diarrhea (staring as early as 12 hours after surgery) and is diagnosed via sigmoidoscopy.

3. Spinal ischemia occurs when the blood supply to the distal spinal cord is compromised, and results in paraplegia. Known as the arteria radicularis magna or the artery of Adamkiewicz, this major blood supply to the distal spinal cord can arise anywhere from T8 to L4 but usually comes off the aorta in the chest. This complication occurs most frequently during ruptured AAAs.

4. Leg ischemia, otherwise known as "trash foot," occurs when debris from the aneurysm embolizes down the leg. A technical problem at a distal anastomosis can also cause leg ischemia.

5. Chylous ascites occurs when the lymphatics are not properly ligated at the time of proximal dissection.

SYMPTOMATIC AND RUPTURED AAAs

The following three clinical presentations are considered life-threatening and surgical emergencies:

1. Patients who present with a painful tender pulsatile abdominal mass;

2. Patients who present with a known AAA and have

abdominal pain, back pain, or a tender AAA;

3. Patients with a pulsatile abdominal mass or known AAA in hypovolemic shock and extremis.

In all of these situations the patient is either leaking from the AAA, or the aneurysm is expanding rapidly or has ruptured. The following needs to be done as expeditiously as possible:

1. Start two large bore IVs;

2. Send a type and cross for blood;

3. Take the patient to the operating room immediately. DO NOT GO TO SONOGRAPHY, ARTERIOGRAPHY, THE INTENSIVE CARE UNIT, OR ANYWHERE BUT THE OPERATING ROOM.

4. The patient is to be prepped and draped while awake, and if time permits, a Foley catheter and central venous pressure line are inserted. Only when the surgeon is ready to make the incision is the patient put to sleep.

5. Control of the ruptured aorta can usually be obtained by clamping the aorta as it enters the abdomen at the diaphragmatic hiatus through the gastrohepatic ligament. An alternative method is to place a large Foley into the rupture and inflate the balloon for temporary tamponade of the bleeding.

AAAs AND COEXISTENT MALIGNANCIES

Rarely, a patient is explored for an AAA and found to have an intraabdominal tumor or vice versa. The best rule of thumb is to operate first on the most life-threatening condition; if neither is immediately life-threatening, do the surgery for which the patient was scheduled. A bowel anastomosis and a vascular operation should not be done at the same time in an elective case.

SUGGESTED READINGS

1. Crawford, E.S., Bush, H.L., Szilagyi, D.E., et al.: Symposium: Prevention of Complications of Abdominal Aortic Reconstruction. Surgery 93:91, 1983.

2. Crawford, E.S., Salva, A.S., Babb, J.W., et al.: Infrarenal Aortic Aneurysms. Ann Surg 193:699, 1981.

3. Estes, J.E.: Abdominal Aortic Aneurysms: A Study of One Hundred and Two Cases. Circulation 2:258, 1950.

4. Szilagyi, D.E., Smith, R.F., Franklin, J., et al.: Contribution of Abdominal Aortic Aneurysmectomy to Prolongation of Life. Ann Surg 164:679, 1966.

5. Whittemore, A.D., Clowes, A.W., Hechtman, H.B., et al.: Aortic Aneurysm Repair: Reduced Operative Mortality Associated with Maintenance of Optimal Cardiac Performance. Ann Surg 192:414, 1980.

6. Cohen, J.R.: Current Concepts for the Pathogenesis of Abdominal Aortic Aneurysms. Perspectives in Vascular Surgery 3(2):103-111, 1990.

Chapter 10

Other Arterial Aneurysms

Several mechanisms have been proposed for the development of arterial aneurysms, including hemodynamic forces acting on the arterial wall, atherosclerosis in the setting of hypertension, congenital defects in the arterial wall, and abnormalities in wall biochemistry as related to the metabolism of collagen. Because multiple aneurysms occur so frequently in the patient with one peripheral aneurysm, many now believe that aneurysm formation is truly a <u>systemic disease</u>, having described it as "<u>aneurysmosis</u>." Clinical evidence that this is a systemic disease includes:

1. Of those patients with a peripheral aneurysm, 80-90% have another aneurysm;

2. Of those patients with a popliteal aneurysm, 80% have another aneurysm, 60% have an abdominal aortic aneurysm, and 50% have bilateral popliteal aneurysms;

3. Of those patients with a femoral aneurysm, 75-90% have another aneurysm;

4. Of those patients with abdominal aortic aneurysms, 20% have popliteal aneurysms;

5. Of those patients with multiple aneurysms, the intervening arteries are frequently much larger than normal and have been termed "<u>arteriomegaly</u>."

Because associated aneurysms are so common in these patients, it is mandatory that the workup include a careful search for other aneurysms by both careful physical examinations and ultrasound of the contralateral extremity and abdominal aorta.

ILIAC ARTERY ANEURYSMS

Isolated iliac aneurysms are relatively rare clinical entities which are usually asymptomatic. The diagnosis is difficult to make prior to the development of symptoms, because of their location in the pelvis. As a result, approximately 60% of these patients first present with rupture of a previously undiagnosed aneurysm. If symptoms do occur, they are usually related to the genitourinary or musculoskeletal systems. A very interesting clinical finding reported in a few of these patients is the presence of a perianal ecchymosis as a result of a contained iliac aneurysm rupture.

The diagnostic test of choice is either an ultrasound or CT scan of the pelvis. All diagnosed iliac aneurysms should be surgically corrected (asymptomatic or symptomatic) by either aneurysmorrhaphy or ligation and bypass grafting. The operative mortality is 52% for those patients repaired emergently (ruptured) and only 5% for those repaired electively.

FEMORAL ARTERY ANEURYSMS

True atherosclerotic femoral aneurysms are also very uncommon. As mentioned above, they are usually associated with other peripheral aneurysms (75-90%) and most often present as asymptomatic pulsatile groin masses. Like popliteal aneurysms, they have a greater tendency to thrombose than to rupture. Treatment is usually aneurysmorrhaphy for both asymptomatic and symptomatic lesions.

POPLITEAL ARTERY ANEURYSMS

The natural history of popliteal aneurysms was first published by Linton in 1949 when he reported that 77% of limbs with popliteal aneurysms followed over an 18-year period were amputated if left untreated. The major reason for limb loss is the high propensity for thrombosis and subsequent severe ischemia.

Popliteal aneurysms are bilateral in 50% of cases and are associated with abdominal aortic aneurysms in 60-70% of cases. As mentioned above, it is mandatory to perform abdominal and contralateral leg ultrasounds as part of the workup.

The diagnostic test of choice is an ultrasound. Arteriography should be done preoperatively to aid in planning reconstruction. Because the end result can be so disastrous if they thrombose (limb loss), all popliteal aneurysms (including small ones greater than 2 cm) should be repaired when diagnosed. The usual treatment is ligation and bypass grafting.

CAROTID ARTERY ANEURYSMS

These are relatively rare clinical entities resulting from atherosclerosis in only 50% of cases. Other cases have resulted from either previous trauma or carotid endarterectomy.

A large number of these patients present with symptoms of cerebrovascular insufficiency (50%), most probably as a result of emboli from the aneurysms. The diagnosis is usually evident by palpation of a pulsatile neck mass, although several cases have involved aneurysms at the origin of the carotid in the chest which are not palpable.

All patients are treated, whether symptomatic or not, by either aneurysmorrhaphy or resection and grafting. Some patients may require intraoperative shunting around the lesion for cerebral ischemia during the repair.

SUBCLAVIAN ARTERY ANEURYSMS

There are rare clinical entities caused by either atherosclerosis, thoracic outlet obstruction, or trauma. Since they occur so infrequently, generalizations about their clinical course are hard to find. Several reports of embolization to the arm and hand have been reported as well as isolated cases of thrombosis and rupture.

The diagnostic test of choice is arteriography, and treatment is by either aneurysmorrhaphy or ligation and bypass grafting.

SPLENIC ARTERY ANEURYSMS

Of all the visceral vessels, the splenic artery most commonly is aneurysmal. The interesting feature of splenic artery aneurysms is their overwhelming predominance among women of childbearing age. They exist most commonly in multiparous females and are usually found incidentally on angiograms done for other reasons.

Pathologically, the lesion is a medial degeneration of the arterial wall and the presence of multiple aneurysms along the course of the splenic artery. Gestational increases in splenic blood flow in conjunction with alteration of estrogen levels during pregnancy are thought to contribute to the selection of the splenic artery as the most common visceral site. Because of the increased splenic blood flow during pregnancy, it is considered mandatory to repair these lesions in pregnant women and women of childbearing age. The mortality from a ruptured splenic artery aneurysm during pregnancy is 68%.

The preferred treatment is resection and repair of the artery, but in many cases the aneurysm is too distal and a splenectomy is required. The actual rupture rate is estimated to be 5-10% for the other patients and is related to the size of the aneurysm such that any aneurysm greater then 2-3 cm and those that are symptomatic should be repaired.

RENAL ARTERY ANEURYSMS

Like splenic artery aneurysms, a majority are found incidentally on arteriograms done for other reasons. They are most commonly found at the renal artery bifurcation and are thought to be related to changes in flow dynamics at the bifurcations. The natural history of these lesions seems to be quite benign except in pregnant women, in whom the rupture rate is higher. They rarely rupture, thrombose, or embolize and are especially stable if less than 2 cm.

Symptoms, when they occur, include hypertension, flank pain, or occasionally hematuria.

The indications for surgery include only pregnant women and patients with coexistent renovascular hypertension. The repair of renal artery aneurysms in patients with coexistent hypertension has not usually cured the hypertension unless high renins were assayed from the aneurysmal kidney.

ANASTOMOTIC ANEURYSMS

The common femoral artery at the site of previous aortofemoral grafting is the most common site for the development of this type of aneurysm. The possible etiologies include degeneration of the native femoral artery, graft manufacturing defect, improper suture placement, and local complications of the procedure such as bleeding or mechanical stress at the end-to-side anastomosis. The most common cause is a suture line dehiscence due to degeneration of the native arterial wall.

The majority of these patients present with asymptomatic

pulsatile groin masses and a history of previous aortofemoral bypass grafting. Usually the diagnosis is evident, but a sonogram is sometimes helpful.

All anastomotic false aneurysms should be repaired if larger than 2 cm. Surgery usually involves resection of the aneurysm including a piece of the graft and placement of an interposition graft.

MYCOTIC ANEURYSMS

The term "mycotic" is actually a misnomer that is used to describe all infected aneurysms despite the fact that almost all are due to bacteria and not fungus.

The sources of infection in the development of these lesions include

1. Intraarterial drug abuse;

2. Penetrating trauma;

3. Septic emboli.

The overwhelming majority of these lesions are currently due to intraarterial drug abuse under contaminated conditions. The clinical picture is usually one of a drug addict with fever and a pulsatile groin mass that is obviously infected. The mass over the femoral artery is usually indurated and cellulitic and may be oozing both pus and blood from the injection site.

Patients should be admitted immediately and placed on intravenous antibiotics after the blood and any obvious pus has been cultured. A good initial regimen should include nafcillin and gentamicin, because the majority of these patients have grown both <u>Staphylococcus</u> <u>aureus</u> <u>and</u> <u>Pseudomonas</u> from their initial wound and blood cultures. A preoperative arteriogram is necessary for planning arterial reconstruction.

With adequate systemic levels of antibiotics on board, the patient should undergo emergent surgery. The most important operative principle includes <u>resection</u> <u>and</u> <u>debridement</u> of all infected artery and surrounding tissues after proximal and distal arterial control are obtained. The proximal and distal artery is ligated and the <u>wound</u> <u>is</u> <u>packed</u> <u>open</u>. The wound is treated with wet to dry dressings and allowed to heal by secondary intention.

Obviously, the extremity will be ischemic with no arterial inflow. The degree of ischemia varies from patient to patient and usually determines the timing of arterial reconstruction. It is best to wait at least 1 week before attempting reconstruction, but in some cases the extremity will not tolerate a significant ischemia time. The reconstruction consists of an "<u>extraanatomical</u>" <u>bypass</u> <u>graft</u> around the area of infection. Usually, synthetic grafts are necessary because of the lack of usable veins in most drug addicts. The grafts should be placed in an area that is relatively inaccessible to the patient, as a majority of these patients will use the graft for further injections. The amputation rate for mycotic aneurysms is 20-25% in most series.

SUGGESTED READINGS

1. Dent, T.L., Lindenauer, M., Ernst, C.B., et al.: Multiple Arteriosclerotic Arterial Aneurysms. Arch Surg 105:338-344, 1972.

2. Feldman, A.J., Berguer, R.: Management of an Infected Aneurysm of the Groin Secondary to Drug Abuse. Surg Gynecol Obstet 157:519-522, 1983.

3. Hobson, R.W., Sarkaria, J., O'Donnell, J., et al.: Atherosclerotic Aneurysms of the Subclavian Artery. Surgery 85:368-371, 1979.

4. Hollier, L.H., Batson, R.R., Cohn, I.: Femoral Anastomotic Aneurysms. Ann Surg 191:715-720, 1980.

5. Johnson, J.R., Ledgerwood, A.M., Lucas, C.E.: Mycotic Aneurysm. Arch Surg 118:577-582, 1983.

6. Linton, R.R.: The Atherosclerotic Popliteal Aneurysm. Surgery 26:41-57, 1949.

7. McCready, R.A., Pairolero, P.C., Gilmore, J.C., et al.: Isolated Iliac Artery Aneurysms. Surgery 93:688-693, 1983.

8. Queral, L.A., Flinn, W.R., Yao, J.S., et al.: Management of Peripheral Arterial Aneurysms. Surg Clin North Am 59:693-706, 1979.

9. Rhodes, E.L., Stanley, J.C., Hoffman, G.L., et al.: Aneurysms of the Extracranial Carotid Arteries. Arch Surg 111:339-343, 1976.

10. Satiani, B., Kazmers, M., Evans W.: Anastomotic Arterial Aneurysms. Ann Surg 192:674-682, 1980.

11. Stanley, J., Fry, W.: Pathogenesis and Clinical Significance of Splenic Artery Aneurysms. <u>Surgery</u> 76:898-909, 1974.

12. Tham, G., Ekelund, L., Herrlin, K., et al.: Renal Artery Aneurysms. <u>Ann Surg</u> 197:348-352, 1983.

13. Vermilion, B.D., Kimmins, S.A., Pace, W.G., et al.: A Review of One Hundred Forty Seven Popliteal Aneurysms with Long Term Follow-up. <u>Surgery</u> 90:1009-1014, 1981.

14. Whitehouse, W.M., Wakefield, T.W., Graham, L.M., et al.: Limb Threatening Potential of Atherosclerotic Popliteal Artery Aneurysms. <u>Surgery</u> 93:694-699, 1983.

Chapter 11

Renovascular Hypertension

The basis for renovascular hypertension lies in an understanding of the <u>renin-angiotensin system</u> control of the blood pressure. The basic pathway is as follows:

1. <u>Renin</u> is an enzyme produced in the juxtaglomerular cells of the afferent arterioles of the kidney and released into the renal veins in response to decreased renal blood flow.

2. Renin acts on a plasma substrate to produce <u>angiotensin I</u>.

3. Angiotensin I is converted to <u>angiotensin II</u> in the pulmonary circulation by an enzyme known as <u>converting enzyme</u>. Converting enzyme can be pharmacologically inhibited by the antihypertensive drug <u>Captopril</u>. Angiotensin II is a very potent vasoconstrictor of arterial smooth muscle in addition to stimulating the secretion of aldosterone from the adrenal cortex. Aldosterone elevates blood pressure by increasing the absorption of sodium and hence water.

In patients with unilateral renal artery stenosis, the blood pressure rises initially in response to renin and the increase in sodium and water retention. Shortly thereafter the opposite kidney will maintain normal fluid balance by excreting the additional volume. Thus, in those patients with unilateral renal artery stenosis, the renin levels remain elevated but volume remains normal, resulting in what is referred to as <u>renin-dependent</u> <u>hypertension</u>. Renin-dependent hypertension is similar to the classic Goldblatt model for unilateral renal artery stenosis in the setting of two kidneys.

In those patients with bilateral renal artery stenosis, renin is produced by both kidneys and the intravascular volume is increased and maintained. Feedback mechanisms result in normal or decresed renin values with high intracellular fluid, resulting in what is referred to as <u>volume-dependent</u> <u>hypertension</u> with bilateral renal artery stenosis. This is similar to the two-kidney Goldblatt model with bilateral renal artery stenosis or unilateral renal artery stenosis in an animal model with only one kidney.

<u>DIAGNOSIS</u>

Patients suspected of hypertension based upon renal artery stenoses should undergo arteriography to establish the presence of renal artery lesions and the extent of involvement on both sides. Renal artery lesions are most often due to atherosclerosis and less commonly due to fibromuscular dysplasia (see below). In the presence of renal artery stenoses, venous sampling of both renal veins and the inferior vena cava near the renal veins is performed for analysis of renin concentrations. The mere presence of a renal artery stenosis does not indicate that the hypertension is based upon the lesion but rather that venous sampling is necessary to help establish the diagnosis. In patients with unilateral renal artery stenosis, a <u>renin ratio</u> of the affected kidney to the opposite kidney of 1.5 or greater is highly suggestive that the stenosis is a functional lesion. The ratio of <u>renal vein renins to systemic values</u> (IVC) of 0.5 or greater is also highly suggestive of a functional lesion. More recently, the Captopril stimulation test is more predictive than renal vein renins in predicting surgical response to renal vascular hypertension.

<u>TREATMENT</u>

The criteria for surgical intervention are continually changing as new drugs are developed to manipulate the renin-angiotensin system. Surgery in older patients is usually reserved for uncontrollable hypertension refractory to maximal medical therapy. Younger patients, especially children, and women of childbearing age with severe hypertension are more aggressively studied in hopes of finding a correctable lesion. Young women with hypertension are very likely to have <u>fibromuscular hyperplasia</u> of the renal arteries as the cause of their hypertension (see below).

Once a functional lesion has been established, surgical procedures to correct the stenosis are varied and include such procedures as aortorenal bypasses, aortic endarterectomies, hepatic-renal artery bypass, and spleno-renal bypass. Balloon dilation of the renal artery of atherosclerotic lesions not involving the renal artery orifice is an excellent therapeutic option with reasonably good results.

FIBROMUSCULAR DYSPLASIA (FMD)

FMD is the second most common type of renal artery lesion and predisposes the renal artery to both stenotic and aneurysmal disease. Different histological types exist, the most common being dysplasia of the media and collagen overgrowth as a result of vasa vasora occlusion.

Radiographically, the lesion has a characteristic appearance of multiple circumferential bands in the middle and distal renal artery. The disease is most common in younger women and may be related to estrogen production. Balloon dilation has been very successful in patients with FMD and has become the treatment of choice, with surgery reserved for those patients unresponsive to dilation.

SUGGESTED READINGS

1. Couch, N.P., Sullivan, J., Crane, C.: The Predictive Accuracy of Renal Vein Renin Activity in the Surgery of Renovascular Hypertension. Surgery 79:70-76, 1976.

2. Dean, R.H., Wilson, J.P., Burko, H., Foster, J.H.: Saphenous Vein Aortorenal Bypass Grafts. <u>Ann</u> <u>Surg</u> 180:469-478, 1974

3. Fry, W.J., Fry, R.E.: Surgically Correctable Hypertension. In <u>Principles</u> <u>of</u> <u>Surgery</u>, edited by S.I. Schwartz, ed 4, pp 1003-1019. McGraw-Hill, New York, 1984.

4. Goldblatt, H.: Hypertension of Renal Origin. <u>Am</u> <u>J</u> <u>Surg</u> 107:21-25, 1964.

5. Novick, A.C., Straffon, R.A., Stewart, B.H., et al.: Diminished Operative Mortality in Renal Revascularization. <u>JAMA</u> 246:749-753, 1981.

6. Skeggs, L.T., Dorer, F.E., Kahn, J.R., et al.: The Biochemistry of the Renin-Angiotension System and Its Role in Hypertension. <u>Am</u> <u>J</u> <u>Med</u> 60:737-748, 1976.

7. Stanley, J.C., Fry, W.J.: Surgical Treatment of Renovascular Hypertension. <u>Arch</u> <u>Surg</u> 112:1291-1297, 1977.

8. Stanley, J.C., Gewertz, B.L., Fry, W.J.: Renal:Systemic Indices and Renal Vein Renin Ratios as Prognostic Indicators in Remedial Renovascular Hypertension. <u>J</u> <u>Surg</u> <u>Res</u> 20:149-155, 1976.

Chapter 12

Aortoiliac Occlusive Disease

Arterial insufficiency of the lower extremities can be categorized into two major groups:

1. Aortoiliac disease affecting the distal aorta, common iliac artery, and external iliac artery or

2. Femoral-popliteal-tibial disease of the arteries of the leg.

Aortoiliac disease is commonly referred to as "<u>inflow</u>" obstruction to the groin, whereas femoral popliteal disease is referred to as "<u>outflow</u>" <u>obstruction</u> with reference to the groin. Both types of disease result in ischemia to the lower extremity, manifested by either claudication, rest pain, or ulceration of the lower extremity.

Chronic arterial insufficiency of the lower extremity is almost invariably due to atherosclerosis (Chapter 3). Although atherosclerosis is a widely systemic disease, its propensity for <u>segmental</u> <u>occlusions</u> within the arterial tree makes it amenable to surgical repair.

Focal lesions of atherosclerosis develop in areas more prone to endothelial injury such as arterial bifurcations or areas of posterior fixation where shearing forces and turbulent flow are the highest. The common sites for these focal lesions causing lower extremity ischemia include the distal aorta, the bifurcation of the common iliac artery, the bifurcation of the common femoral artery, and the superficial femoral artery at the adductor canal.

A basic understanding of the <u>physics</u> <u>of</u> <u>blood</u> <u>flow</u> is essential to the understanding of arterial occlusive disease. Blood flow, like any circuit, is broadly described by the formula

$$\underline{FP} = \underline{P/R}, \quad \text{where} \quad \underline{F} = \text{flow}, \quad \underline{P} = \text{pressure, and}$$
$$\underline{R} = \text{resistance.}$$

Flow is thereby directly proportional to the pressure and inversely proportional to the resistance within the circuit.

Flow within any actual artery with a stenotic lesion is specifically governed by the Poiseuille equation:

$$\underline{Q} = \underline{(p1-p2)(pi)(r)(4)} / \underline{(m)(8)(l)}$$

where $\underline{Q}$ = flow, $\underline{p1}$-$\underline{p2}$ = pressure differential, $\underline{r}$ = radius, $\underline{m}$ = viscosity, and $\underline{l}$ = length.

Thereby, to a large extent, flow is determined by the radius of the arterial lumen and the length of the intraluminal stenosis. In addition, sequential arterial obstructions within the same artery provide resistance to flow such that each obstruction is essentially additive.

Arterial stenoses and obstruction enhance the development of collateral vessels from existing smaller arteries. Small arterial branches above and below the obstruction anastomose to provide an autogenous bypass around the lesion. Collaterals usually take time to develop, and their presence is evidence of a long-standing obstructive lesion. Patients who present with acute obstructions have not had time to develop adequate collaterals and thereby present with a much more severe degree of ischemia. Collaterals are the most important compensatory mechanism for atherosclerotic vascular disease but, unfortunately, can only partially compensate for an occlusion or severe stenosis.

THE NATURAL HISTORY OF CLAUDICATION OF THE LOWER EXTREMITIES

Intermittent claudication is a benign process in the overwhelming majority of patients. The natural history of claudication was first reported by Boyd, where he followed 440 patients with intermittent claudication for 5-15 years. The important results of this study are as follows:

1. Only 7.2% of patients required a major amputation in 5 years.

2. Only 12% required a major amputation at 10 years.

3. Only 38% were alive at 10 years, and 22% of the entire group were alive at 15 years.

The second important study was reported by Imparato, where 104 claudicators were arteriogrammed and followed (Fig. 12.1). The results of this study were as follows:

1. Claudication remained stable or improved in 80% of patients.

2. Only 5.8% of the entire group went on to develop gangrene.

3. Twenty-five percent of the entire group ultimately required surgical therapy.

Based on these studies, only 5-10% of patients with claudication will actually develop gangrene and thereby be at risk of losing their limbs. Given these data, the majority of claudicators can be treated conservatively and only undergo surgery for disabling claudication (see below).

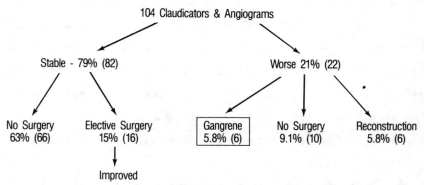

Figure 12.1.   Fate of 104 claudicators. (From Imparato, A.M., Kim, G.E., Crowley, J.G.: Intermittent Claudication: Its Natural Course. Surgery 78:795, 1975.)

Patients who have <u>rest</u> <u>pain</u>, <u>ulcerations</u>, or <u>gangrenous</u> changes in their feet have a completely different prognosis. They are considered to be in the "<u>threatened</u> <u>limb</u> <u>loss</u>" category and are at the end stage of their disease. <u>All</u> of these patients will go on to <u>lose</u> <u>the</u> <u>extremity</u> without surgical correction.

Clinical Presentation

The history of patients with aortoiliac disease is invariably one of <u>hip,</u> <u>thigh,</u> <u>or</u> <u>buttock</u> <u>claudication</u> frequently described as "tiredness" when walking which is relieved by rest. Some of these patients will have claudication in their calves. Another very important historical finding is one of <u>impotence</u> in males. Examination of these patients is usually remarkable for an <u>absence</u> <u>of</u> <u>femoral</u> <u>pulses</u> or markedly diminished <u>femoral</u> pulses with <u>bruits</u>.

<u>Doppler</u> <u>measurements</u> of patients with peripheral arterial disease are an <u>essential</u> part of the physical examination (see Chapter 4, Fig. 4.1 for how a Doppler works). Accurate recording of Doppler pressures is critical for the hospital stay and subsequent long-term follow-up. The easiest and most standard measurement is the <u>ankle/brachial</u> <u>index</u> (<u>ABI</u>). Measurements are made with the blood pressure cuff at the ankle. With the cuff inflated, placing the Doppler over the posterior and dorsalis pedis

arteries, the systolic pressure is recorded. An arm pressure is also recorded and the ratio computed. In normal patients, the ABI should be 1.0. In claudicators, the ABI is usually 0.6 to 0.9, whereas in patients with either rest pain or ulcerations the index is usually less then 0.5. Diabetics frequently have artificially elevated ABIs as a result of calcified tibial vessels that require more pressure to compress. The ABI should be recorded before and after surgery and then followed. Any drop in pressure after surgery should be aggressively worked up for possible graft stenosis. Despite the ABI, no patient should be denied an arteriogram for threatened limb loss in hopes of finding a correctable lesion.

Treatment

As discussed above, the overwhelming majority of patients with claudication should be treated conservatively with vigorous medical therapy which includes

1. Stop smoking. This cannot be stressed enough to patients with peripheral vascular disease, as smoking is the major cause for progression of disease.

2. A vigorous exercise program where the patients are advised to "walk through" the claudication. This means that when the pain starts they should try to exercise or walk a little further each time.

3. Patients should be worked up for hyperlipidemia and treated appropriately for high lipids, triglycerides, or cholesterol.

4. Diabetics should have their diabetes tightly controlled.

On a vigorous medical exercise program over 85% of patients with claudication will actually improve their walking distance and never require surgery.

Indications for surgery in patients with arterial insufficiency of the lower extremities include

1. Disabling claudication whereby the patient cannot perform his day-to-day activities necessary for work or a relatively normal existence;

2. Rest pain;

3. Gangrene or ulceration;

4. Leriche's syndrome. Described in 1940 by Leriche, this is comprised of specific symptoms stemming from the gradual occlusion of the terminal aorta. The five specific manifestations of the early stages of the disease include

   a. Sexual impotence;

   b. Extreme fatigue of the legs with exercise;

   c. Atrophy of the leg muscles;

   d. Presence of trophic changes of the feet;

   e. Pallor of the legs.

The early stages of Leriche's syndrome are well tolerated, but most patients progress to severe disabling claudication.

Those patients with threatened limb loss should be admitted to the hospital as soon as possible and angiogrammed. During the interim they should be kept at <u>bed rest</u> in the reverse <u>Trendelenburg</u> position with <u>broad spectrum</u> <u>antibiotics</u> started until culture results are obtained. The reverse Trendelenburg position will improve distal flow and significantly improve the patient's discomfort during the interim between admission and surgery. A <u>sheepskin</u> blanket under the feet and a cradle to keep the bed covers off the feet are important adjuncts to patient comfort.

Surgery for patients with aortoiliac disease consists of three broad options:

1. In good-risk patients, the operation of choice is an <u>aortobifemoral</u> <u>graft</u>.

2. In patients with unilateral iliac artery occlusion but good flow into the opposite groin, <u>a</u> <u>femoral-femoral crossover</u> <u>bypass</u> is an excellent option and can be done safely under local anesthesia if necessary.

3. In patients considered poor surgical risks but who absolutely need revascularization, an "<u>extraanatomical</u>" bypass can be performed. This is usually via an <u>axillobifemoral</u> graft, thus avoiding the need for a large intraabdominal procedure.

Preparation for aortic surgery as discussed in Chapter 8 should include

1. Mild bowel prep;

2. Perioperative antibiotics;

3. Arterial line and Swan-Ganz catheter the night before surgery.

Postoperative care in these patients should include close monitoring of the pedal pulses and nasogastric decompression of the stomach until the ileus resolves.

Results of aortobifemoral grafting for patients with occlusive disease of the lower extremity have been excellent, with patency rates from 85 to 95% at 5 years. Results of axillobifemoral grafts are usually not as good, with patency rates of 70-75% at 5 years. Results of femoral-femoral bypasses have been excellent, with patency rates of 80-85% in most series.

The role of <u>percutaneous</u> <u>transluminal</u> <u>angioplasty</u> <u>(balloon dilation)</u> has become very prominent for isolated iliac artery stenosis (see Chapter 14). Balloon dilation involves placement of an arterial catheter across the stenosis and inflating a balloon to dilate the lesion from within the artery. Results have been poor in most infrainguinal arteries, however, with isolated iliac artery stenosis, patency rates for balloon angioplasty range from 80 to 90% at 5 years.

<u>SUGGESTED</u> <u>READINGS</u>

1. Bernhard, V.M.: The Management of Chronic Occlusive Arterial Disease Affecting the Lower Extremities. In <u>Vascular Surgery</u>, edited by R.B. Rutherford, ed 1, pp 487-496. W.B. Saunders Co., Philadelphia, 1977.

2. Brewster D.C., Darling, R.C.: Optimal Methods of

Aortoiliac Reconstruction. Surgery 84:739-747, 1978.

3. Brief, D.K., Brener, B.J., Alpert, J., et al.: Crossover Femoralfemoral Grafts Followed Up Five Years or More. Arch Surg 110:1294-1299, 1975.

4. DeBakey, M.E.: The Current Status of the Leriche Syndrome. Surg Rounds 20-30, April 1980.

5. Delaurentis, D.A., Friedmann, P., Wolferth, C.C., et al.: Atherosclerosis and the Hypoplastic Aortoiliac System. Surgery 83:27-37, 1978.

6. Imparato, A.M., Riles, T.S.: Peripheral Arterial Disease. In Principles of Surgery, edited by S.I. Schwartz, ed 4, pp 901-910. McGraw-Hill, New York, 1984.

7. Jones, A.F., Kempczinski, R.F.: Aortofemoral Bypass Grafting. Arch Surg 116:301-305, 1981.

8. Kadir, S., White, R.I., Kaufman, S.L., et al.: Long Term Results of Aortoiliac Angioplasty. Surgery 94:10-14, 1983.

9. LoGerfo, F.W., Johnson, W.C., Corson, J.D., et al.: A Comparison of the Late Patency of Axillobilateral Femoral and Axillounilateral Femoral Grafts. Surgery 81:33-40, 1977.

10. Padberg, F.T., Hobson, R.W., Lynch, T.G. et al.: Assessment of Aortoiliac Insufficiency. Contemp Surg 24:39-45, 1984.

11. Palmaz, J.C., Carson, S.N., Hunter, G., et al.: Male Hypoplastic Infrarenal Aorta and Premature Atherosclerosis. Surgery 94:91-94, 1983.

Chapter 13

Femoropopliteal Occlusive Disease

The most common site of occlusion for patients presenting with claudication of the lower extremity is in the superficial femoral artery at the <u>adductor</u> <u>canal</u> (<u>Hunter's</u> <u>canal</u>). At least 50-60% of patients with intermittent claudication will have an occlusive lesion at this site. Patients with threatened limb loss (rest pain or ulceration) will invariably have another lesion such that collaterals are inadequate to provide enough flow for tissue viability. This second lesion is usually at the profunda femoris takeoff, distal popliteal, or the tibial/peroneal arteries. It is important to recognize the great importance of the <u>profunda</u> <u>femoris</u> <u>artery</u> (deep femoral) as the major flow to the lower extremity when the superficial artery is occluded. The profunda femoris collaterizes with the geniculate arteries around the knee to provide inflow into the distal popliteal artery and the tibial/peroneal arteries.

Claudication of the lower extremity is classically described as pain in the calves when ambulating which is relieved by rest. It is usually quantified in the number of blocks the patient can walk without having to stop. Patients with rest pain have pain in their feet (not in the calf), usually across the forefoot, most prominent at night, relieved by sleeping with their feet in the dependent position (hanging over the side of the bed).

Physical examination is most remarkable for a palpable femoral pulse with no palpable pulses below the groin. Ankle/brachial indexes usually range from 0.6 to 0.9 in claudicators and less than 0.5 in patients with threatened limb loss (see Chapter 12). Trophic changes of arterial insufficiency include thickening of the nails, loss of hair of the lower part of the leg, and shiny skin. Ulceration and gangrene usually start at the most distal toe tips and progress proximally.

<u>TREATMENT</u>

The overwhelming majority of patients with claudication require only medical management, which includes no smoking, vigorous exercise, stopping beta-blockers, tight diabetic control, and correction of hyperlipidemias (see Chapter 12 for the natural history of the claudicator and Fig. 12.1). In a select group of patients with isolated superficial femoral artery stenosis, laser-assisted balloon angioplasty or atherectomy are other therapeutic options (see Chapter 14).

Patients with either severe disabling claudication or threatened limb loss are considered surgical candidates. Surgical options depend on the location of the lesion in relation to the knee. Patients can be categorized into two treatment groups:

1. Patients with disease limited to above the knee that can be helped with an above-knee femoral-popliteal bypass or

2. Patients with disease below the knee requiring a distal bypass to the politeal artery below the knee, tibial-arteries, or pedal arteries.

Patients with above knee occlusions should undergo above-knee femoral-popliteal bypasses with saphenous vein or polytetrafluoroethylene (PTFE) (Gortex). The 5-year patency rates for threatened limb loss with above-knee femoral-popliteal bypasses are 75-80% with a limb salvage rate of 85-95%. The 5-year patency for claudicators with above-knee bypasses is 85-90% with no limb loss (Table 13.1).

The best results for patients who require bypasses to the below knee popliteal artery, the tibial arteries, or the pedal arteries are obtained with autogenous vein. The saphenous vein is usually the graft of choice, but other autogenous veins such as the lesser saphenous vein or arm veins have proven to be excellent alternatives. The results of below-knee bypasses are compared in Table 13.1.

There is a continuing debate as to the operation of choice when using autogenous tissue in the lower extremities; reversed saphenous vein or the saphenous vein _in situ_ technique. With the in situ technique, the saphenous vein is left in its native bed and the valves are made incompetent with a valve cutter (valvulatome or stripper). The advantages of the in situ technique over the reverse technique are

1. The large end of the vein is sewn to the large common femoral artery, and the small end of the vein is used in the smaller distal anastomsis. This provides for a greater _compliance_ _match_, a major cause of graft failure in the reversed technique. Compliance mismatch in reversed veins causes myointimal hyperplasia and graft stenosis.

2. The majority of the vein is never mobilized; thus, its native nutrient supply is never disrupted and the intima is less frequently disrupted.

3. Because the small end of the vein is used for the distal anastomosis, there is a much greater vein utilization rate. Many of the reversed veins were abandoned because the distal vein was too small for the larger proximal anastomosis.

TABLE 13.1

	5-Year Patency	Limb Salvage
Fem-pop above-knee claudication	85-90%	
Fem-pop above-knee limb salvage	75-80%	85-90%
Fem-tib limb salvage	85%	92%

SYMPATHECTOMY

Sympathectomies were frequently performed 10-20 years ago for patients with peripheral vascular disease. They are occasionally used today as adjuncts to vascular reconstruction. The procedure involves division and removal of the sympathetic chain with 3-5 ganglia on the affected side. The operation disrupts all sympathetic tone to the peripheral arterioles. The result is maximal dilation of small arterioles and collaterals, providing increased blood flow to the skin and subcutaneous tissues. Sympathectomies do not increase blood supply to muscle groups. The end result is a warmer foot that may relieve some of the rest pain and occasionally help in healing of small ulcerations. Unfortunately, because of the severity of the preexisting occlusive disease, the small vessels are already maximally dilated and sympathectomy provides little improvement.

The Smithwick test can be used as a reliable guide to patient selection. The test is performed by elevating the ischemic leg for a short period of time to produce maximal tissue anoxia and vasodilation. When the leg is returned to the dependent position, capillary refilling should occur within 20-30 seconds if adequate collaterals are present. If vasodilation and capillary refilling do occur within this period, then the patient should have a favorable response to sympathectomy. Patients without this response probably have insufficient arterial and capillary reserve to benefit from the procedure.

THE DIABETIC FOOT

Diabetics have an increased susceptibility to atherosclerotic vascular disease and infection within their lower extremity. This susceptibility has been blamed on "small vessel disease" or "microangiopathy" inherent to diabetics, although evidence is still lacking to support these theories. Despite this debate, there is no question that diabetics are different than other patients with atherosclerosis in that the distribution of disease primarily involves the tibial/peroneal arteries.

Diabetic neuropathy rather than microvascular disease is actually the primary cause of lesions of their feet. Patients sustain trauma to their feet without being aware and develop ulcerations of the metatarsal heads and heel. Infected ulcerations with subsequent osteomyelitis result in a significant foot infection.

Patients with diabetes should be ultimately compulsive about foot care and see a physician at the earliest sign of trouble. Patients should be given the following instructions about foot care:

1. Inspect the feet daily, looking for calluses, red spots, ulcerations, or infection of the foot and between the toes.

2. Wear adequately fitting shoes that fit well around the balls of the feet and do not crowd the toes.

3. The feet should be kept warm and clean at all times and moisturized with cream to avoid cracks in the skin.

Lanolin should be applied daily.

4. Foot care, especially clipping of the toe nails, should be done by a qualified podiatrist.

Cigarette smoking should be absolutely prohibited in any diabetic, as it accelerates the atherosclerosis. Any sign of infection in the diabetic foot requires immediate hospital admission, bed rest, and broad spectrum I.V. antibiotics. Patients with an infection that does not clear within several days, ulcerations, or rest pain should undergo angiography and vascular reconstruction.

Diabetics with reconstructable lesions do just as well as nondiabetics with similar disease in terms of graft patency and limb salvage. Diabetics should never be written off as having unreconstructable disease until an arteriogram is obtained, and they should be offered the same surgical options as other patients, with expectation of as good results for limb salvage.

SUGGESTED READINGS

1. Brewster, D.C., LaSalle, A.J., Robison, J.G., et al.: Factors Affecting Patency of Femoropopliteal Bypass Grafts. Surg Gynecol Obstet 157:437-442, 1983.

2. Kacoyanis, G.P., Whittemore, A.D., Couch, N.P., Mannick, J.A.: Femorotibial and Femoroperoneal Bypass Vein Grafts. Arch Surg 116:1529-1534, 1981.

3. Karmody, A.M., Leather, R.P., Shah, D.M., et al.: Peroneal Artery Bypass: A Reappraisal of Its Value in Limb Salvage. J Vasc Surg 1:809-816, 1984.

4. Kaufman, J.L., Whittemore, A.D., Couch, N.P., Mannick, J.A.: The Fate of Bypass Grafts to an Isolated Popliteal Artery Segment. Surgery 92:1027-1032, 1982.

5. Lally, M.E., Johnston, W., Andrews, D.: Percutaneous Transluminal Dilation of Peripheral Arteries: An Analysis of Factors Predicting Early Success. J Vasc Surg 1:704-709, 1984.

6. Leather, R.P., Powers, S.R., Karmody, A.M.: A Reappraisal of the In Situ Saphenous Vein Arterial Bypass: Its Use in Limb Salvage. Surgery 86:453-461, 1979.

7. LoGerfo, F.W., Coffman, J.D.: Vascular and Microvascular Disease of the Foot in Diabetics. Implications for Foot Care. N Engl J Med 311:1615-1618, 1984.

8. Mannick, J.A.: Femoral-Popliteal and Femoral-Tibial Reconstructions. Surg Clin North Am 59:581-596, 1979.

9. Perry, M.O., Hays, R.J.: Lumbar Sympathectomy as an Adjunct in the Management of Arterial Occlusive Disease of the Lower Extremity. Clin Med 19-22, March 1974.

10. Tiefenbrun, T., Beckerman, M., Singer, A.: Surgical Anatomy in Bypass of the Distal Part of the Lower Limb. Surgery 141:528-533, 1975.

11. Whittemore, A.D., Clowes, A.W., Couch, N.P., Mannick, J.A.: Secondary Femoropopliteal Reconstruction. Ann Surg 193:35-42, 1981.

Chapter 14

Alternative Techniques for the Treatment of Vascular Occlusive Disease

In the last 10 years, there has been an explosion in technological advancements in an effort to circumvent the need for surgical intervention for the treatment of occlusive arterial disease. These developments include the use of lasers, balloon angioplasty, arterial stents, atherectomy devices, and intraarterial angioscopy. Using surgical procedures as the gold standard for long-term excellent results, none of the new therapies to date have come close to achieving the same results as surgical intervention. However, improvements in technology may make these therapies more viable alternatives within the next several years.

<u>BALLOON ANGIOPLASTY</u>

Balloon angioplasty is a procedure whereby a balloon catheter is passed through an arterial lesion and the lesion is cracked open with a balloon by inflation of the balloon. The success of balloon angioplasty is dependent on several factors:

1. The indication for the procedure; claudication versus limb salvage;

2. The site of the lesion; common iliac, external iliac, or

femoro-popliteal;

3. The severity of the lesion stenosis versus occlusion;

4. Run-off; good or poor;

5. The number of sites dilated; one, two, or more;

6. The presence of diabetes;

7. The occurrence of complications.

Five-year results of balloon angioplasty are dependent on these factors, with a large diversion of results depending on the individual case. The best results with balloon angioplasty are in the claudicator with a common iliac artery stenosis and good run-off. The percent success in this scenario is 63% five-year patency. The worst scenario is the patient who presents for limb salvage with a femoro-popliteal occlusion with poor run-off, where the five-year patency is 10%. In general, most authors feel that balloon angioplasty alone should be reserved for common iliac artery lesions in the claudicator. Balloon angioplasty alone in lesions below the inguinal ligament have had poor results in the long-term, and most specialists are not advising balloon angioplasty alone for infrainguinal lesions.

LASER-ASSISTED BALLOON ANGIOPLASTY

Lasers are currently used as an adjunct to balloon angioplasty. With these devices, laser energy is converted to heat in the range of 200-400°C which locally melts or vaporizes the atheromatous obstruction. Current "hot-tipped" laser angioplasty catheters are used to bore a channel through the arterial obstruction or to make the arterial stenosis wider, followed by balloon angioplasty of the lesion. An alternative to the hot-tip technology has been the development of controlled free light laser angioplasty systems whereby the end of the catheter actually emits a percentage of the energy directly to the atheromatous plaque. Development is underway for target-specific laser angioplasty with identification of specific tissue for lasing using fluorescence patterns to identify the target atheromatous tissue.

Unfortunately, to date the results of laser-assisted angioplasty have been poor. Currently the major limitation of laser-assisted angioplasty is the length of the occluded segment to be traversed. Laser recannulation is most successful for lesions 15 cm in length or shorter in the common iliac or superficial femoral arteries. Results with tibial vessels have been extremely disappointing.

Current studies indicate that overall patency for successful procedures of the superficial femoral artery are 55% at three months, 38% at six months, and 11% in 12 months. Most vascular specialists agree that laser angioplasty has a very limited role in advanced peripheral vascular disease but may provide an alternative in small subsets of patients such as high-risk patients with threatened limb loss and medical conditions that would prohibit surgery.

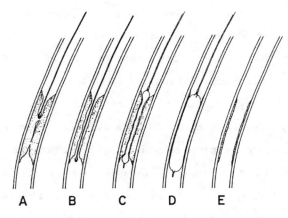

Figure 14.1. Schematic diagram of laser assisted balloon angioplasty (A, B) Recanalization of arterial occlusion by passage of the activated "hot-tipped" laser. (C, D) Balloon dilation of the recanalized segment. (E) Idealized result. (Reproduced with permission, Journal of Vascular Surgery, Ref. 2.)

ATHERECTOMY CATHETERS

As discussed above, the major limitations with laser-assisted balloon angioplasty and balloon angioplasty alone have been the poor results because of the uncontrolled damage that a balloon does and the failure to achieve success in long and complex lesions. A newer approach has been the use of atherectomy catheters, which is the selective removal of atheromatous plaque from atherosclerotic vessels while leaving the media intact done percutaneously.

Many atherectomy devices are available. The three most commonly used are

1) Simpson Peripheral Atherectomy Catheter. This catheter contains a cutting device and retrieval chamber for the debris, in addition to an opposing balloon. The balloon engages the longitudinal opening into the atheroma and fixes the unit to the atherosclerotic vessel, after which a hand-held motor-driven device slices the plaque, pushing it into the collection chamber.

2) The Kensey Atherectomy Device is a drive shaft with a tip on an electric motor that rotates approximately 2000 rpm. The rotating tip is designed to pulverize atheromatous tissue and produce little damage to the elastic tissue of the blood vessel.

3) The Rotablator is a catheter-tipped device that rotates at high speed through which the rotary bur with diamond chips within it cuts through the atheromatous plaque.

The Simpson and Rotablator thus far seem relatively safe, whereas the Kensey catheter seems to have a higher risk of perforation. The Kensey catheter, however, is designed for totally occluding lesions, whereas the Simpson and Rotablator are best suited for vessels with high-grade stenoses rather than total occlusion. The use of all three devices leaves a lumen that is relatively smooth compared with percutaneous balloon angioplasty with minimal flaps and dissections.

The results, however, of all these devices are very preliminary to date, and there are no available data on the long-term success. Most of these devices are still in clinical trials, so that their place in the armamentarium of the vascular surgeon is yet to be fully defined.

ANGIOSCOPES

Like other endoscopic tools, the angioscope is used for direct visualization of blood vessels and bypass grafts. Its major advantage is that it allows immediate detection and correction of technical errors and deficiency during surgery. Other uses may include intraluminal visualization during procedures such as thrombectomy, embolectomy, and atherectomy and angioplasty. Because of the ongoing blood that accumulates within the lumens, irrigation with balanced salt solutions is used to keep the field clear and the angioscope tip free of obstruction.

The angioscope in the proper hands is a valuable adjunct to the vascular surgeon, however, its value compared with completion angiography during distal bypass is yet to be defined.

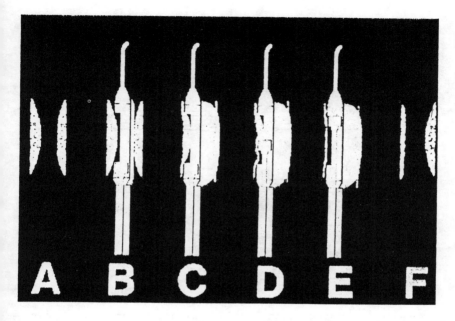

Figure 14.2. Diagram of the Simpson atherectomy procedure.
(A) The lesion before atherectomy. (B) Atherectomy catheter
in position across the lesion. (C) The balloon support
inflated. (D) The cutter advanced. (E) The specimen trapped
in the housing. (F) The balloon deflated and the catheter
removed. (Reproduced with permission, WB Saunders, Ref. 15.)

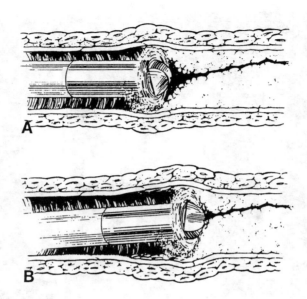

Figure 14.3. During recanalization with the Kensey catheter, the rotating cam seeks out the path of least resistance, tracking from the normal arterial lumen (A) into the reduced lumen in the diseased segment (B). (Reproduced with permission, The Radiological Society of North America Inc., Ref. 16.)

VASCULAR STENTS

Intravascular metallic stents are currently under development as a way to prevent the early occlusion or re-stenosis after transluminal balloon angioplasty or laser assisted angioplasty. Most of these are expandable stainless steel mesh stents that could be implanted by balloon expansion at the site of the stenosis. These devices are delivered over an angioplasty balloon to the site of the stenosis and are expanded by inflation of the balloon. They maintain the expanded state after the balloon is deflated and removed. Use of stents is currently under clinical trials, and whether or not restenosis will be significantly inhibited by the use of stents is yet to be seen. To date, the use of stents in the coronary circulation in humans has been poor at best. Complications include acute vessel closure, thrombosis, dissection, inadequate expansion, and migration of the stent. Further development of this area may lead to exciting new therapeutic options for the future.

SUGGESTED READINGS

1. Johnston, K.W., Rae, M., Hogg-Johnston, S.A., et al.: 5-Year Results of a Prospective Study of Percutaneous Transluminal Angioplasty. Ann Surg 206:403-413, 1987.

2. White, R.A., White, G.H.: Laser Thermal Probe Recanalization of Occluded Arteries. J Vasc Surg 9:598-608, 1989.

3. Seeger, J.M., Abela, G.S., Silverman, S.H., et al.:

Initial Results of Laser Recanalization in Lower Extremity Arterial Reconstructions. J Vasc Surg 9:10-17, 1989.

4. Snyder, A.O., Wheeler, J.R., Gregory, R.T., Gayle, R.G., Mariner, D.R.: The Kensey Catheter: Preliminary Results with a Transluminal Atherectomy Tool. J Vasc Surg 8:541-543, 1988.

5. Ahn, S.S.: Peripheral Atherectomy. Semin Vasc Surg 2(3):143-154, 1989.

6. Palmaz, J.C., Richter, G., Noeledge, G., et al.: Intraluminal Stents in Atherosclerotic Iliac Artery Stenosis: Preliminary Report of a Multicenter Study. Radiology 168:727-731, 1988.

7. Ahn, S.S., Auth, D., Marcus, D.R., Moore, W.S.: Removal of Focal Atheromatous Lesions by Angioscopically Guided High-Speed Rotary Atherectomy. J Vasc Surg 7:292-300, 1988.

8. Wright, J.G., Belkin, M., Greenfield, A.J., Guben, J.K., Sanborn, T.A., Menzoian, J.O.: Laser Angioplasty for Limb Salvage: Observations on Early Results. J Vasc Surg 10:29-38, 1989.

9. Blebea, J., Ouriel, K., Green, R.M., Fiore, W.M., Welch, E.L., Svoboda, J.J., Balaji, M.R.: Laser Angioplasty in Peripheral Vascular Disease: Symptomatic versus Hemodynamic Results. J Vasc Surg 13:222-230, 1991.

10. Grundfest, W.S., Litvack, F., Glick, D., et al.: Intraoperative Decisions Based on Angioscopy in Peripheral Vascular Surgery. Circulation 78(suppl I):I-13-I-17, 1988.

11. Miller, A., Campbell, D.R., Gibbons, G.W., et al.: Routine Intraoperative Angioscopy in Lower Extremity Revascularization. Arch Surg 124:604-608, 1989.

12. Cikrit, D.F., Becker, G.J., Dalsing, M.C.: Early Experience with the Palmaz Expandable Intraluminal Stent in Iliac Artery Stenosis. Ann Vasc Surg 5:150-155, 1991.

13. Hinahora, T., Robertson, G.C., Selmon, M.R., et al.: Percutaneous Atherectomy: The Simpson Atherectomy Catheter, In Endovascular Surgery, WB Saunders, Philadelphia, edited by Moore, W.S., Ahn, S.S., pp 310-322, 1989.

14. Kensey, K.R., Nash, J.E., Abrahams, C., et al.: Recanalization of Obstructed Aarteries with a Flexible, Rotating Catheter-Tip. Radiology 165:387-389, 1987.

Chapter 15

Mesenteric Vascular Disease

The diagnosis of mesenteric vascular insufficiency is one of the most difficult clinical diagnoses to make. In most cases the diagnosis can only be made with a high index of suspicion and angiography in the setting of minimal physical findings. The gastrointestinal tract is supplied by the celiac, superior mesenteric (SMA), and inferior mesenteric arteries with a rich collateral network between the three vessels. Most patients are asymptomatic with occlusion of two of the three arteries and only become symptomatic when the remaining one vessel becomes stenotic or occludes. The most common cause is atherosclerosis at the origin of the vessels.

ACUTE MESENTERIC INSUFFICIENCY

As in other types of acute insufficiency, the cause can be either an embolus or thrombosis. Most commonly, the cause is an embolus to the SMA originating from the heart in a patient with atrial fibrillation or a recent myocardial infarction and mural thrombus. The classic diagnostic triad for those patients with an embolus includes

132

1. <u>Acute</u> <u>abdominal</u> <u>pain</u>;

2. <u>Significant</u> <u>cardiac</u> <u>disease</u>;

3. <u>Acute</u> <u>gastrointestinal</u> <u>emptying</u>.

The most common <u>risk</u> <u>factors</u> for those patients with an arterial embolus are <u>atrial</u> <u>fibrillation</u> and a history of taking <u>digoxin</u>.

Those patients with acute thrombosis usually

1. Have severe coexistent atherosclerotic disease;

2. Have a history of previous chronic abdominal pain (intestinal angina);

3. Are older;

4. Have a recent history of a low cardiac output event (i.e., shock).

<u>Digoxin</u> is commonly taken by those patients with both types of acute insufficiency. The role of digoxin has not been clearly defined and may be related to its direct vasoconstrictor effect on the smooth muscle of the mesenteric blood supply, or it may be that patients with poor cardiac output and poor ventricular function are more susceptible to this disease and happen to also be receiving digoxin.

In both types of insufficiency, the pain is usually sudden in onset, intermittent at first, and progressing on to continuous severe pain. Patients may present with vomiting or diarrhea which may be bloody, before or after the onset of pain. The most important part of the presentation in both entities is the <u>relative</u> <u>lack</u> <u>of</u>

abdominal tenderness in relation to the severity of the abdominal pain. Significant physical findings occur after transmural necrosis of the bowel wall occurs, at which point it is usually too late to save the patient.

DIAGNOSIS

The diagnostic test of choice is angiography of the mesenteric circulation, including lateral views of both the celiac axis and SMA. In patients where the issue of mesenteric insufficiency has been raised, early angiography is the only key to improved patient survival. Many of these patients are very ill intensive care unit patients, making their physicians reluctant to move them to angiography. This tendency to wait is the most common major therapeutic error. If the diagnosis is suspected, angiography must be done immediately so that revascularization can be performed before too much bowel necrosis.

Angiographically, emboli usually lodge at the branch of the middle colic artery with less extensive involvement of the origin of the proximal SMA. Spasm usually occurs distal to the embolus with resultant ischemia to the entire small bowel and proximal colon. Because collaterals are usually not present, the time to bowel infarction is quick. Thrombosis usually occurs at the origin of the artery with more extensive distal thrombosis. Since patients with thrombosis usually have long-standing prior ischemia, collaterals are more frequently present so that the time to bowel infarction may be longer.

Other diagnostic clues in helping to raise the index of suspicion are an elevated white count with a left shift, persistent metabolic acidosis, and relatively normal abdominal x-rays.

TREATMENT

If the angiogram demonstrates mesenteric insufficiency then <u>papaverine</u> should be started immediately to help dilate the vasospastic distal circulation. Papaverine is infused at a constant rate via the angiographic catheter directly into the mesenteric circulation (30-60 mg/hour). Subsequent surgical treatment depends upon whether the diagnosis is an embolus or thrombosis. For those patients with an embolus, an <u>emergent</u> <u>embolectomy</u> should be performed with restitution of distal blood supply. For those patients with a thrombosis, a proximal stenosis in the SMA is almost always implicated. In this situation an <u>aortomesenteric</u> <u>bypass</u> is necessary to reestablish adequate flow. Only after blood flow is reestablished is the bowel evaluated for viability and resection performed. At the time of the original procedure the decision to perform a "<u>second</u> <u>look</u>" operation should be made to reevaluate the viability of the bowel. Any bowel with questionable viability should be left in until the second look to preserve as much bowel length as possible.

CHRONIC INTESTINAL INSUFFICIENCY

This is a rare entity involving insufficient blood flow to the small intestine, resulting in "intestinal angina." The symptoms result in postprandial abdominal pain beginning 10-60 minutes after a meal, usually abating in 1-4 hours. All patients have a fear of food, resulting in a significant weight loss at the time of presentation.

The only remarkable physical finding is the presence of an abdominal bruit in a majority of patients. As in acute mesenteric ischemia, suspicion must be high because the only diagnostic test is arteriography. Occlusion of at least two of the three mesenteric vessels with stenosis of the third is necessary to make the diagnosis. Patients with a wide open celiac or SMA are unlikely to have this disease.

Treatment usually consists of revascularization of the SMA via a vein graft off the aorta or an aortic endarterectomy of both the SMA and the celiac axis.

NONOCCLUSIVE MESENTERIC INFARCTION

This entity involves diffuse intestinal necrosis without a proximal embolus or thrombosis. It usually results from a severe low cardiac output state as in any type of severe shock (i.e., sepsis, cardiogenic, hypovolemic). Leukocytosis, fever, and hemoconcentration are several common findings in these types of cases. Angiograms reveal no proximal lesion with a low flow state to the small bowel and colon. The treatment is to correct the underlying cause of the low cardiac output in conjunction with intraarterial papaverine. Resection is usually not possible because of the extensive involvement of the bowel, resulting in a mortality rate of 80-90%.

MEDIAN ARCUATE LIGAMENT SYNDROME

Whether this entity actually exists is still questioned by many authorities of gastrointestinal vascular disease. The syndrome results from compression of the celiac axis by the median arcuate ligament of the diaphragm.

Patients are usually thin females, 40-60 years of age, with a history of weight loss and abdominal pain when eating. The pain is less severe than that of classic intestinal angina. On physical examination, upper abdominal bruits are invariably heard.

The diagnostic test of choice is lateral arteriography, which reveals compression of the celiac axis by the median arcuate ligament.

Treatment consists of division of the median arcuate ligament and the celiac plexus.

SUGGESTED READINGS

1. Adams, J.T.: Abdominal Wall, Omentum, Mesentery. In Principles of Surgery, edited by S.I. Schwartz, ed 4, pp 1431-1441. McGraw-Hill, New York, 1984.

2. Bergan, J.J., Conn, D.J., Yao, J.S.: Revascularization in Treatment of Mesenteric Infarction. Ann Surg 182:430-438, 1975.

3. Boley, S., Sprayregan, S., Siegelman, S., Veith, F.: Initial Results from an Aggressive Roentgenological and Surgical Approach to Acute Mesenteric Ischemia. Surgery 82:848-855, 1977.

4. Boley, S.J., Bergan, J.J, Williams, L.F., Zuidema, G.: Acute Mesenteric Vascular Occlusion Symposium. Cont Surg 22:125-164, 1983.

5. Ottinger, L.W.: The Surgical Management of Acute Occlusion of the Superior Mesenteric Artery. Ann Surg 188:721-731,1978.

6. Stanley, J., Fry, W.: Median Arcuate Ligament Syndrome. Arch Surg 103:252-258, 1971.

7. Stoney, R., Ehrenfeld, W., Wylie, E.: Revascularization Methods in Chronic Visceral Ischemia Caused by Atherosclerosis. Ann Surg 186:468-476, 1977.

8. Williams, L.F.: Vascular Insufficiency of the Intestines. Gastroenterology 61:757-777, 1971.

Chapter 16

Portal Hypertension

ANATOMY AND PHYSIOLOGY OF THE HEPATIC CIRCULATION

The liver receives blood from both the hepatic artery and portal vein. The portal vein anatomically begins behind the pancreas where the superior mesenteric and splenic veins join. The left gastric vein or coronary vein enters the portal vein at its origin, and it is important in the pathophysiology of portal hypertension. The portal vein subsequently divides into right and left branches.

The hepatic artery is one of the major branches of the celiac axis and provides approximately 25% to 35% of the blood flow to the liver, although it is responsible for 50% of the liver's oxygen supply. The portal vein provides the remaining portion of the blood supply to the liver.

Pathophysiology of Portal Hypertension

Portal hypertension is defined as an abnormal elevation in the portal venous system pressure. Resistance to portal flow resulting in portal hypertension is divided into three major subcategories:

1. Presinusoidal - portal vein thrombosis and schistoso-miasis;

2. Sinusoidal - cirrhosis;

3. Postsinusoidal - Budd-Chiari (obstructive hepatic veins).

139

The major cause of portal hypertension in children is portal vein thrombosis, and frequently it is a result of umbilical lines and catheters. Schistosomiasis is the most common cause of presinusoidal portal hypertension in the world, given its endemic occurrence in third world countries. In the United States, cirrhosis as a result of alcoholism is the most common cause of portal hypertension (over 90% of cases). The Budd-Chiari syndrome (hepatic vein thrombosis) is the most common cause of postsinusoidal portal hypertension, which usually occurs in hypercoagulable patients.

As a result of the increase of portal vein pressure collaterals between the portal and systemic venous system develop. The major sites of connection between the portal and venous circulation are as follows (Fig. 16.1):

1. Periumbilical, resulting in caput Medusa;

2. retroperitoneal plexes, resulting in retroperitoneal bleeding from the veins of Retzius;

3. hemorrhoidal veins, resulting in severe hemorrhoids;

4. left coronary vein off of the portal vein connecting with the azygos in the system thorax, resulting in marked dilation of esophageal veins and gastric veins, which results in esophageal and gastric varices.

The most significant clinical problem is esophageal and gastric varices resulting in upper gastrointestinal bleeding.

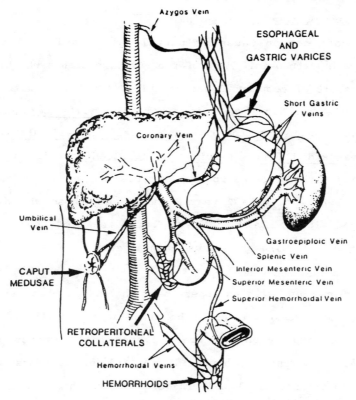

Figure 16.1.   Sites of portal-systemic collateralization. (Reproduced with permission, Essentials of General Surgery Williams & Wilkins.)

Upper Gastrointestinal Bleeding

The most common cause of portal hypertension in this country is cirrhosis. Most of the 90% of patients who bleed as a result of esophageal varices bleed from sites within 2 cm of the esophageal-gastric junction. Fifty percent of patients who bleed from esophageal varices rebleed within one year and die as a result of that bleeding episode. Of patients with known esophageal varices who have not bled, 30% will bleed within 2 years, and 79% of those who bleed are dead within 1 year. Ninety-four percent of those with or without bleeding are dead within 5 years.

Diagnosis and Treatment

Any patient with an upper gastrointestinal bleed with a history of alcoholism should be immediately stabilized and then undergo upper gastrointestinal endoscopy. Interestingly enough, approximately 50% of patients with upper gastrointestinal hemorrhages with esophageal varices have bleeding from other sites including diffuse gastritis, peptic ulcer disease, and Mallory-Weiss tears.

Other signs and symptoms suggesting that the patient has chronic alcoholic cirrhosis are the presence of palmar erythema, gynecomastia, spider angiomata, caput Medusa, ascites, and a palpable liver and/or spleen. Treatment for acute esophageal bleeding includes the following:

1. Intravenous fluids, type and cross match blood;

2. Gastric lavage with a large bore nasogastric tube;

3. Admission to an intensive care unit;

4. Oral lactulose to induce diarrhea and decrease the absorption of ammonia;

5. Possibly systemic pitressin, which is used to lower portal pressure and decrease inflow to the portal venous system;

6. If the above measures do not stop the bleeding, then mechanical means are used. The Sengstaken-Blakemore tube can be used to compress effectively the bleeding varices while blood and fluid is administered and coagulation abnormalities are corrected (Fig. 16.2);

7. Endoscopic sclerotherapy is now the preferred the treatment for bleeding esophageal varices and can be performed acutely.

Patients are not considered surgical candidates unless they are failures of sclerotherapy. It is difficult to define failure; however, most physicians agree that at least three attempts at adequate sclerotherapy should be attempted.

Surgical Therapy for Portal Hypertension

Operations for decompression of the portal system have been an interest to surgeons for many years. The basis for the surgery is to decompress the portal system and to alleviate the high pressure within the portal system to stop the bleeding esophageal varices. In the past, one bleeding episode was an indication for surgical intervention; however, with the advent of aggressive endoscopic sclerotherapy, surgery is now reserved for sclerotherapy failures. More recently, patients with significant end-

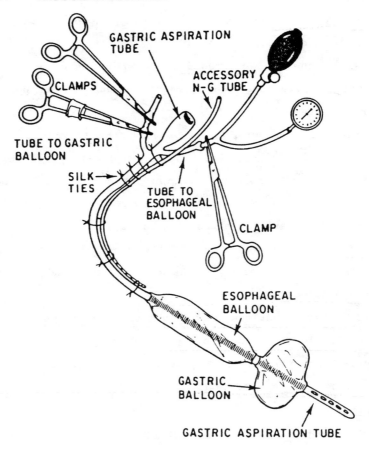

Figure 16.2. Sengstaken-Blakemore tube. (Reproduced with permission, _Essentials of General Surgery_, Williams & Wilkins.)

stage liver disease have had liver transplants as a possible surgical treatment for the disease. The results of transplantation in cirrhotics is not yet available, but if patients have stopped drinking for at least six months prior to surgery then transplantation may be the best alternative for patients with end-stage liver disease. Certainly patients with idiopathic cirrhosis may be good candidates for liver transplantation as opposed to portal decompressive surgery.

Several types of portal decompressive surgery exist including the following (Fig. 16.3):

1. Portacaval shunts

   a. <u>End-to-side</u> <u>portacaval</u> <u>shunt</u> - in this operative procedure the portal vein is completely divided and the distal end of the portal vein is sewn to the side of the inferior vena cava, providing a total rerouting of the portal blood into the inferior vena cava. The major problem with this type of shunt is the high incidence of encephalopathy, since none of the portal flow can be decontaminated and detoxified with resultant high levels of systemic ammonia. <u>End-to-side portacaval shunts do work well for stopping esophageal variceal bleeding and effectively decompressing the portal circulation</u>.

   b. <u>Side-to-side</u> <u>portacaval</u> <u>shunt</u> - this operative procedure is similar to the above; however, the side of the portal vein is sewn to the side of the inferior vena cava thereby theoretically not directing all of the portal flow away from the liver. However, in reality in patients with severe portal hypertension, the flow may actually be directed away from the liver in addition to rerouting portal flow because of the high resistance of the distal portal circulation. Like the above procedure, the incidence of encephalopathy is extremely high.

c. H-graft portacaval shunt - similar to the above procedure, instead of a side-to-side anastomosis a large diameter Gortex or Dacron graft is placed from the side of the portal vein to the side of the inferior vena cava, with the resulting effects similar to those with the side-to-side portacaval shunt.

d. Small-diameter H-graft (Sarfeh shunt) - in this procedure a 8 or 10 mm Ringed Gortex graft is placed between the side of the portal vein and the inferior vena cava, which theoretically provides enough decompression to the portal system to stop bleeding but not enough to redirect all portal flow, with a reported lower incidence of encephalopathy than the above-mentioned three procedures.

e. The distal splenal renal shunt (Warren shunt) - this shunt is completely different than the central decompression shunts listed above. This is the only portal systemic shunt that preserves portal flow to the liver. The operation consists of anastomosing the distal splenic vein to the left renal vein and disconnecting the portal circulation from the varices by ligating the coronary vein. Varices are then selectively decompressed through the short gastric veins into the splenic vein and then into the renal vein into the systemic circulation. Encephalopathy rates following distal shunts have been reported to be significantly lower than those with nonselective essential shunts.

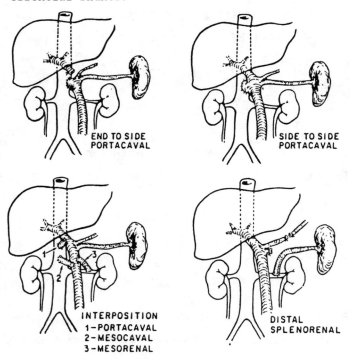

Figure 16.3. Surgical portal-systemic shunts. (Reproduced with permission, Essentials of General Surgery, Williams & Wilkins.)

Predicting Operative Mortality in Patients with Portal
Hypertension

The Child's classification is the traditional
classification system used to approximate operative
mortality for shunt surgery (Table 16.1).

TABLE 16.1

CHILD'S CLASSIFICATION

CRITERIA	GOOD RISK (A)	MODERATE RISK (B)	POOR RISK (C)
Serum bilirubin (mg/100 ml)	<2.0	2.0-3.0	>3.0
Serum albumin (mg/100 ml)	>3.5	3.0-3.5	<3.0
Ascites	None	Easily controlled	Not easil controlle
Encephalopathy	None	Minimal	Advanced
Nutrition	Excellent	Good	Poor

SUGGESTED READINGS

1.   Abouna, G.M., Baissony, H., Al-Nakib, B.M., Menkarios,
      A.T., Silva, O.S.G.: The Place of Sugiura Operation for
      Portal Hypertension and Bleeding Esophageal Varices.
      Surgery 101(1):91-98, 1987.

2.   Warren, W.D., Henderson, J.M., Millikan, W.J., et al.:

Distal Splenorenal Shunt versus Endoscopic Sclerotherapy for Long-term Management of Variceal Bleeding. Ann Surg 203(5):454-462, 1986.

3. Cello, J.P., Grendell, J.H., Crass, R.A., Weber, T.E., Trunkey, D.D.: Endoscopic Sclerotherapy versus Portacaval Shunt in Patients with Severe Cirrhosis and Acute Variceal Hemorrhage. New Engl J Med 316(1):11-15, 1987.

4. Rikkers, L.F., Burnett, D.A., Volentine, G.D., Buchi, K.N., Cormier, R.A.: Shunt Surgery versus Endoscopic Sclerotherapy for Long-term Treatment of Variceal Bleeding. Ann Surg 206(3):261-270, 1987.

5. Sarfeh, I.J., Rypins, E.B., Mason, G.R.: A Systematic Appraisal of Portacaval H-Graft Diameters. Ann Surg 204(4):354-363, 1986.

6. Burroughs, A.K., Hamilton, G., Phillips, A., Mezzanotte, G., McIntyre, N., Hobbs, K.: A Comparison of Sclerotherapy with Staple Transection of the Esophagus for the Emergency Control of Bleeding from Esophageal Varices. New Engl J Med 321(13):857-862, 1989.

7. Henderson, J.M., Millikan, W.J.: Portal Hypertension. Am J Surg 160(1):4-138, 1990.

Chapter 17

Thoracic Outlet Syndromes

Thoracic outlet syndromes refer to neurovascular problems resulting from compression at the thoracic outlet by either cervical ribs or fibromuscular bands. Symptoms can be related to <u>compression</u> <u>of</u> <u>either</u> <u>the</u> <u>brachial</u> <u>plexus,</u> <u>subclavian</u> <u>artery,</u> <u>or</u> <u>subclavian</u> <u>vein</u>.

The major anatomical variation in these patients is usually the presence of a <u>cervical</u> <u>rib</u> (Fig. 17.1). The other important anatomical relationship of the region is the course of the subclavian artery behind the <u>scalenus</u> <u>anticus</u> <u>muscle</u> (Fig. 17.1).

CLINICAL PRESENTATION

The vast majority of patients with thoracic outlet syndrome present with intermittent, progressive <u>neurological</u> symptoms. The C8-T1 nerve roots of the brachial plexus are most often compressed against the cervical rib as the brachial plexus exits from the thoracic outlet, thus affecting the distribution of the ulnar nerve most frequently. Patients frequently complain of pain, paresthesias, numbness, and weakness in the neck, shoulder, or hand.

Symptoms of arterial insufficiency occur rarely and include pain, claudication, and coolness of the hand or arm.

Venous symptoms occur very infrequently and are the

result of subclavian vein thrombosis. Symptoms include varicosities, cyanosis, and edema of the arm.

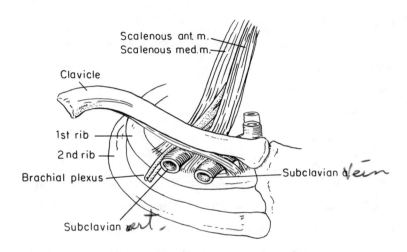

Figure 17.1. Anatomy of the thoracic outlet.

PHYSICAL FINDINGS

The <u>Adson</u> <u>test</u> is classically described for arterial symptoms of thoracic outlet compression but actually can only be documented in a very small percentage of cases. The test is performed with the neck in extension, arms at the side, chin towards the symptomatic side, and deep inspiration while the radial pulse is palpated. All of these maneuvers cause tension on the scalenus anticus. A positive test is a diminution or loss of the radial pulse during inspiration in this position.

A complete neurological examination is the most important diagnostic tool. Findings in the distribution of the ulnar nerve include weakness of the intrinsic hand muscles, atrophy of the hand muscles, and weakness of the triceps.

Blood pressure should be measured in both extremities and the hand and fingers carefully examined for signs of ischemia or gangrene. Bruits over the subclavian artery should be documented, as well as any sign of venous hypertension.

DIFFERENTIAL DIAGNOSIS AND DIAGNOSTIC TESTING

The differential diagnosis includes any tumor of the thoracic outlet or cervical spine, cervical disk disease at the C8-T1 interspace, carpal tunnel syndrome, arthritis of the cervical spine, atherosclerosis of the subclavian artery, or trauma to any part of the neurovascular bundle.

The most important initial studies are a chest x-ray and cervical spine films, followed by specific testing depending on the presenting symptoms. Unfortunately the majority of neurological tests, including nerve conduction studies and electromyography, have not been useful and are no longer recommended. On occasion a myelogram may be necessary to rule out a C8-T1 herniated disk. Angiography may be useful for the rare patient presenting with either arterial or venous compromise.

The most reliable diagnostic tool is a high index of suspicion after a detailed history and physical examination in the patient with a cervical rib on x-ray.

TREATMENT

The majority of patients can be managed conservatively regardless of the symptoms. Conservative therapy includes an exercise program to strengthen the shoulder girdle, cervical halters, and patient education to keep the shoulders from drooping and the arm from hyperabduction.

The indications for surgery include disabling pain resulting in the inablility to work or function daily or significant loss of function of the extremity.

The mainstay of surgical treatment involves resection of the first cervical rib via an axillary approach with simultaneous division of the scalenus anticus and medicus muscles. In those patients with arterial insufficiency, the lesion is resected and replaced with a graft with simultaneous rib resection. Patients with venous occlusion may be helped with rib resection and concomitant venous thrombectomy and/or intravenous urokinase into the involved extremity.

SUGGESTED READINGS

1. Imparato, A.M., Riles, T.S.: Peripheral Arterial Disease. In Principles of Surgery, edited by S.I. Schwartz, ed 4, pp 936-941. McGraw-Hill, New York, 1984.

2. Kelly, T.R: Thoracic Outlet Syndrome. <u>Ann</u> <u>Surg</u> 190:657-662, 1979.

3. Roos, D.B.: Thoracic Outlet Syndrome. <u>Rocky</u> <u>Mt</u> <u>Med</u> <u>J</u>, 64:49, 1967.

4. Roos, D.B.: Thoracic Outlet and Carpal Tunnel Syndromes. In <u>Vascular</u> <u>Surgery</u>, edited by R.B. Rutherford, ed 1, pp 605-621. W.B. Saunders Co., Philadelphia, 1977.

5. Scher, L.A., Veith, F.J., Haimovici, H., et al.: Staging of Arterial Complications of Cervical Rib: Guidelines for Surgical Management. <u>Surgery</u> 95:644-648, 1984.

6. Urschel, H.C., Razyuk, M.A.: Management of Thoracic Outlet Syndrome-Current Concepts. <u>N</u> <u>Engl</u> <u>J</u> <u>Med</u> 286:1140, 1972.

Chapter 18

Amputations

The most frustrating part of vascular surgery is the inability to save part of an extremity, resulting in an amputation. Amputations are performed in vascular surgery for either gangrene or irreversible, painful ischemia not amenable to vascular reconstruction.

Vascular patients undergoing amputations invariably have severe coexistent systemic atherosclerotic disease. This is reflected by an operative mortality of 13% for above-knee (AK) and below-knee (BK) amputations. One-half of this extremely high mortality for these relatively quick extraperitoneal procedures is directly attributable to heart disease. The 3-year survival of patients undergoing major amputations (AK and BK) is only 50% and drops to 30% at 5 years, again a reflection of the severe coexistent cardiovascular disease.

The rehabilitation rates (ability to walk independently) for all patients undergoing major amputations are as follows:

BK	66%
AK	36%
BILATERAL BK	45%
or BK + AK	
BILATERAL AK	11%

Excluding those patients chronically debilitated or demented prior to amputation and considering those patients who were candidates for a prosthesis, the rehabilitation rates are as follows:

BK	90%
AK	76%
BILATERAL BK or MIXED	62%
BILATERAL AK	40%

THE AMPUTATION DECISION

The decision for amputation in the presence of dry gangrene or ulceration should never be made until all possibilities of arterial reconstruction have been ruled out. Patients with dry gangrene of the toes are unlikely to heal toe amputations without arterial reconstruction.

Diabetes has little effect on the healing rate or revision rate of amputation, so diabetics should be subjected to the same criteria for selection of amputation site as nondiabetics.

Once the decision to amputate has been made, the appropriate level for amputation must be decided. The majority of surgeons base their decision on clinical features such as the proximal extension of the gangrene or infection, skin appearance (rubor), and temperature of the proposed site. The critical decision is usually whether the amputation should be below the knee or above the knee. Much more accurate testing is now available to predict healing at the amputation site; however, the clinical availability of these tests is usually restricted. For instance, excellent correlation has been found between the level of amputation and skin blood flow as determined by xenon-133 injection. Xenon skin flow measurements of 2.6 ul/min/100 gm of tissue or greater at the proposed level of amputation is 97% accurate in predicting healing; however, most clinicians do not have this test available to them. Doppler measurements have not been as accurate as xenon skin blood flow, but in some series a pressure of 70 mm Hg or greater at the calf has been associated with a healing rate of 97% for BK amputations.

PREOPERATIVE PREPARATION

Adequate tissue levels of the appropriate antibiotics, based upon culture and sensitivity reports, are the most important aspect in preoperative preparation. For patients with wet gangrene or abscesses, broad spectrum antibiotics including gram-negative coverage should be instituted until sensitivity results are available. The overall majority of these infections are <u>polymicrobial</u>.

In patients with wet gangrene or abscesses requiring emergent operation for control of sepsis, all of the infected tissue is removed at the first operative procedure with delay of the formal amputation. This might include partial foot or complete foot amputation followed by a formal below-knee amputation 3-5 days later after the patient's local sepsis has been cleared. Many patients will have abscesses or collections of the ventral foot requiring emergent incision and drainage with delay of the formal amputation. After the infection has cleared the appropriate level of amputation is then determined and the amputation is performed.

In those patients with severe ischemia above the knee, it may be necessary to establish adequate arterial inflow into the femoral artery at the groin to heal an AK amputation.

<u>DIGITAL AMPUTATIONS</u>   (Fig. 18.1)

The majority of patients undergoing digital amputations have diabetes with <u>diabetic peripheral neuropathy</u> and <u>osteomyelitis</u> of the phalanges.

The important aspects of the perioperative care in patients with toe amputations include

1. 7-10 days of perioperative antibiotics;

2. Strict bed rest for 1-4 weeks;

3. No weight bearing for 2-6 weeks;

4. Suture removal at 3-6 weeks.

For those patients requiring amputation of the great toe, preservation of the first metatarsal head (ball of the foot), whenever possible, is critical for subsequent foot balance and walking.

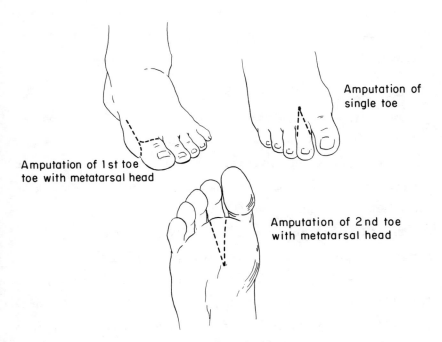

Figure 18.1. Incisions for toe amputations.

(From   Sizer J.S.,   Wheelock, F.C.: Digital Amputation in Diabetic Patients. Surgery, 72:980, 1972.)

TRANSMETATARSAL AMPUTATIONS (Fig. 18.2)

Ischemia or gangrene limited to several toes or the forefoot can be treated by transmetatarsal amputation. In the majority of cases, a localized infection in the ventral aspect of the foot can be incised and drained prior to amputation. After local control of the infection, antibiotics, and dressings, the patient is returned to the operating room 7-10 days later for the definitive amputation.

Postoperatively, the patient is kept at strict bed rest for 1-2 weeks with no weight bearing on the extremity for 4-6 weeks.

SYME'S AMPUTATION

This type of amputation is rarely done for peripheral vascular disease because rarely does arterial disease involve just the distal part of the foot. It involves removal of the entire foot including the calcaneus, with preservation of the entire tibia (Fig. 18.2).

Syme's amputations are classically performed for trauma, tumors, or congenital anomalies of the foot. They are usually done in males because the prosthesis is bulky and cosmetically inferior to BK prostheses. Weight is borne primarily on the distal tibia, but some weight bearing is transferred to the tibial condyles and patellar tendon by the prosthesis.

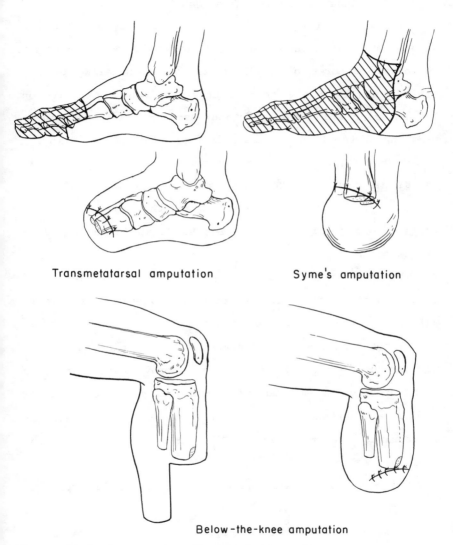

Transmetatarsal amputation   Syme's amputation

Below-the-knee amputation

Figure 18.2. Lower extremity amputation sites.

BELOW KNEE AND ABOVE KNEE AMPUTATIONS

BK amputations are the most common type of major amputations for ischemia and gangrene. The most important technical features of a BK amputation is beveling of the tibial tuberosity such that no pressure ischemia results on the anterior skin flap. Meticulous hemostasis and gentle handling of the flaps is essential for good wound healing.

AK amputations heal more frequently and are especially useful in the older bedridden patient who will never be ambulatory. AK amputations are done with a circumferential incision and equal flaps, placing the scar in the mid-line of the stump.

The prostheses for BK and AK amputations are significantly different. BK prostheses are much easier to walk on for the following reasons:

1. Balance function is better with the knee joint in place.
2. There is less of an increase in energy expenditure with BK prostheses. BK amputations require approximately a 10% increase in energy expenditure, while an AK prosthesis requires as much as a 67% increase in basal energy requirements.
3. With a BK prosthesis there is circumferential support. Weight is equally distributed so that 30% of the weight is borne by each tibial condyle and 40% of the weight is borne by the patellar tendon.

4. With an AK prosthesis the weight bearing is noncircumferential and completely borne by the ischium. In addition, the corset that keeps the AK prosthesis in place rotates commonly. Sitting is more difficult with the AK prosthesis and an artificial knee joint.

PHYSIOLOGICAL AMPUTATIONS

On rare occasions, a patient is severely ill and becomes a prohibitive surgical risk because of concomitant systemic disease or sepsis. In this setting, a medical amputation can be performed by freezing the leg with an arterial tourniquet in place. The involved extremity is packed in ice-filled plastic bags and a thigh tourniquet is placed with a continuous pressure gauge at 600 mm Hg. The physiological amputation prevents further seeding from the infected extremity and essentially autoamputates the leg. If the patient survives the initial insult, 24-48 hours later the patient is taken to the operating room for a guillotine amputation which is closed at a future date. It is important to protect the skin of the opposite viable extremity from touching the ice-filled bags and becoming damaged.

GENERAL PRINCIPLES

The following are general surgical principles that are important in any amputation:

1. Control of localized infection prior to excision of tissue.

2. Intravenous antibiotics for 1-2 weeks if possible in an attempt to sterilize the lymphatics prior to elective amputation.

3. Minimal handling of the skin flaps during surgery is critical to subsequent flap viability (no skin forceps).

4. Meticulous hemostasis is extremely important for flap viability.

5. Drainage whenever there is a possibility of collections.

6. Monofilament, nonabsorbable sutures are used for skin closure and are removed 4-6 weeks after surgery.

SUGGESTED READINGS

1. Couch, N. P., David, J.K., Tilney, N.L., et al.: Natural History of the Leg Amputee. Am J Surg 133:469-473, 1977.

2. Effency, D.J., Lim, R.C., Schecter, W.P.: Transmetatarsal Amputation. Arch Surg 112:1366-1370, 1977.

3. Hicks, L., McClelland, R.N.: Below Knee Amputations for Vascular Insufficiency. Am Surg 239-243, 1980.

4. Kacy, S.S., Flye, M.W.: Factors Affecting the Results of Below the Knee Amputation in Patients with and without Diabetes. Surg Gynecol Obstet 155:513-518, 1982.

5. Lee, B.Y., Madden, J.L., Thorden, W.R., et al.: Syme's Amputation Revisited. Cont Surg 22:31-40, 1983.

6. Moore, S.M.: Lower Extremity Amputation for Peripheral Vascular Disease. Surg Rounds, 16-22, Jan. 1982.

7. Moore, W.S., Henry, R.E., Malone, J.M., et al.: Prospective Use of Xenon Xe 133 Clearance for Amputation Level Selection. <u>Arch Surg</u> 166:86-88, 1981.

8. Sizer, J.S., Wheelock, F.C.: Digital Amputation in Diabetic Patients. <u>Surgery</u> 72:980-989, 1972.

Chapter 19

Vasculitis and Vasospastic Syndromes

BUERGER'S DISEASE

Buerger's disease is an inflammatory process that affects moderate-sized arteries and often nearby veins and nerves. The result is known as <u>thromboangiitis</u> <u>obliterans</u>, often associated with a superficial phlebitis and occasionally neuritis. Buerger's disease is <u>always</u> <u>associated</u> <u>with</u> <u>heavy</u> <u>smoking</u>.

Characteristically the tibial and peroneal arteries are most often involved while the vessels proximal to the popliteal are remarkably normal. The inflammatory process frequently involves the adjacent vein, producing a <u>migratory</u> <u>superficial</u> <u>recurrent</u> <u>phlebitis</u> that rarely involves the larger veins.

Pathological examination reveals lymphocytes and a dense fibrous reaction around the involved arterial wall, with occasional extension to the neighboring nerve and vein.

The usual patient is male, 20-40 years old, with a clinical course marked by periods of acute exacerbations associated with smoking. Claudication may be severe with rapid progression to rest pain, ulceration, and limb loss if smoking is not stopped. Remissions will usually occur after the patient stops smoking. Buerger's disease also affects the upper extremity and must be considered in the differential diagnosis of patients with upper extremity arterial insufficiency and finger loss.

Physical examination will reveal severe changes of arterial insufficiency and on occasion a superficial phlebitis. An arteriogram will confirm the classic pattern of "corkscrewing" and multiple segmental occlusions of the smaller arteries with very poor runoff. The proximal arteries are usually normal in marked contrast to the severe distal disease.

The natural history of these patients is quite poor compared with patients with routine atherosclerosis. There is a three times higher mortality from cardiovascular disease, with an amputation rate of 20-30% at 10 years. Treatment is usually limited to conservative measures, most important of which is cessation of smoking. Most patients are not reconstructable, but on occasion a sympathectomy may help to relieve some of the symptoms.

TAKAYASU'S DISEASE

Takayasu's disease is a nonspecific arteritis involving the aortic arch and major arch vessels. It occurs primarily in younger Oriental women.

Pathologically, the arteritis involves the adventitia, with fibrosis of the media and proliferation of the intima causing stenosis and finally obstruction. Symptoms are usually referable to the involved arch vessels. Carotid lesions cause signs of cerebral ischemia, subclavian lesions cause ischemia to the arms, and aortic stenosis causes hypertension.

The disease has a malignant progression such that the majority of patients are dead in 5 years. There is no known therapy.

RAYNAUD'S DISEASE

Raynaud's phenomenon is classically described as episodic, reversible, vasospastic ischemia of the fingers and occasionally the toes. The attack is a "triphasic" sequence of pallor, cyanosis, and reactive hyperemia. Blanching of the fingers and hand when exposed to cold is the most important historical clue.

It is an idiopathic disorder, but recent evidence exists that the defect may be an altered adrenergic receptor in the platelets which responds to stimuli by intense vasospasm. The disease is not curable, but palliative measures can be of help. Therapeutic measures are directed at control of the primary disease or inciting agents.

The usual history is that of a young woman with cold, painful fingers associated with paresthesias and pallor alternating with rubor. Physical exam will reveal ischemic hands and fingers, frequently with ulceration of the finger tips. The disease is primarily limited to the hand and fingers but can affect the nose, cheeks, and ears. The diagnosis can be confirmed by exposing the hands to cold and witnessing the fingers blanch. In 10-30 minutes the fingers will become cyanotic and then turn red from reactive hyperemia.

The differential diagnosis includes lupus, scleroderma, thoracic outlet syndrome, Buerger's, and atherosclerotic emboli to the fingers. Workup should include an arch arteriogram, chest x-ray, and rib films.

Therapy should be directed at controlling the inciting agent or disease with such measures as abstinence from smoking, avoiding exposure to the cold, avoiding stressful stimuli, and wearing loose-fitting gloves. Sympathectomies may be helful in the occasional patient with severe disease. Medical treatment may include intraarterial injection of such vasodilators as reserpine, guanethidine, methyldopa, or tolazoline. Nifedipine, 10 mg, three to four times a day has been found to be particularly helpful in certain subsets of patients with Raynaud's disease.

ACROCYANOSIS

Acrocyanosis is a vasospastic disorder characterized by cold cyanotic hands and feet that are not painful. It is differentiated from Raynaud's by the lack of blanching and no evidence of chronic arterial insufficiency. Acrocyanosis is a constant cyanotic condition as opposed to the alternating cycle of Raynaud's.

The pathophysiology of the condition is an alteration of arteriole tone with chronic constriction and slow blood flow. The slow rate of flow results in a disassociation of the bound hemoglobin and subsequent cyanosis.

The usual clinical presentation is that of a young woman with <u>cold</u>, <u>blue</u> <u>hands</u> <u>and</u> <u>fingers</u> that are made worse with exposure to cold but never have normal color in the affected area.

Treatment consists of conservative measures of avoiding exposure to the cold, or occasionally, sympathectomy.

<u>LIVEDO RETICULARIS</u>

Livedo reticularis is a vasospastic condition characterized by <u>reddish-blue</u> <u>mottling</u> of the skin of the lower extremity, usually made worse with exposure to cold. It is always present and may occur in the upper extremity. Cosmesis is the major complaint of most patients, with little disability.

The pathophysiology is a rare vasospasm or obstruction of the arterioles in the skin of the affected area.

Treatment consists of avoidance of cold, and on rare occasion, sympathectomy.

<u>ERYTHROMELAGIA</u>

Erythromelalgia is a rare disorder characterized by <u>painful</u> <u>burning</u>, <u>itching</u>, and <u>tingling</u> <u>of</u> <u>the</u> <u>lower</u> <u>leg</u> <u>and</u> <u>foot</u> as the <u>environmental</u> <u>temperature</u> <u>increases</u>. There is usually a critical temperature at which the syndrome begins. Patients are quick to learn that cold water can help to abort an attack, and they avoid increases in temperature by wearing open shoes, avoiding foot coverings, and staying in cool environments.

The diagnosis is usually evident by history and physical exam during a provoked attack by warming the skin. Pulses are usually normal while the skin is bright red and warm during an attack. Such drugs as aspirin or methysergide have had variable success in controlling the attacks.

TABLE 19.1

Comparison of Vasospastic and Vasculitis Syndromes Location

	Population at risk	Inciting Agent	Response	Location
	Sex Age			
Buerger's	M 20-40	Smoking	Inflamm.	Tib/per art
Takayasu's	F 20-40	?	Inflamm.	Aortic arch
Raynaud's	F 20-40	Cold Stress Smoking	1. Blanching 2. Cyanosis 3. Rubor	Hands/ fingers
Acrocyanosis	F 20-40	Cold	Cold/blue	Hands/ fingers
Livedo reticularis		Cold	Reddish-bluish mottling	Lower leg
Erythromelagia		Warmth	Burning, red	Lower leg/ foot

SUGGESTED READINGS

1. Imparato, A.M., Riles, T.S.: Peripheral Arterial Disease. In Principles of Surgery, edited by S.I. Schwartz, ed 4, pp 961-964, McGraw-Hill, New York, 1984.

2. Keenan, E.J., Porter, J.M.: Alpha Adrenergic Receptors in Platelets from Patients with Raynaud's Syndrome. Surgery 94:204-209, 1983.

3. Memon, A.S.: Raynaud's Vasospasm. Hosp Pract, 141-149, May 1983.

4. Patrick, G.B.: An Approach to Vasculitis Syndromes. Hosp Pract, 47-65, Jan 1982.

5. Reddi, H.T.: Thromboarteritis Obliterans and/or Buerger's Disease in South India. A Review of 70 Cases. Int Surg 59:555, 1974.

6. Scully, R.E., Mark, E.J., McNeely, B.U.: Weekly Clinicopathological Exercises-Case Presentation-Takayasu's Arteritis. N Engl J Med 305:1519-1524, 1981.

7. Volkman, D.J., Mann, D.L., Fauci, A.S.: Association between Takayasu's Arteritis and a B-Cell Alloantigen in North Americans. N Engl J Med 306:464-465, 1982.

8. Wessler, S.: Buerger's Disease Revisited. Surg Clin North Am 49:703, 1969.

Chapter 20

Arteriovenous Fistula

Arteriovenous fistulae (AVFs) are abnormal connections between a peripheral artery and vein that are classified as either congenital or acquired lesions.

<u>CONGENITAL</u> <u>ARTERIOVENOUS</u> <u>FISTULA</u>

These lesions are one type of abnormality that can occur in the <u>embryological</u> maturation of the vascular system. They are present at birth but may not be recognized until later in development. The clinical manifestations of these lesions vary tremendously between patients, depending on the site and extensiveness of the lesion. They occur most frequently on the extremity and may involve the skin, subcutaneous tissue, muscle, and bone.

As a result of the abnormal arteriovenous connection, more blood than usual goes to the affected extremity. With an increase in flow, more blood is shunted through the fistula, resulting in <u>venous</u> <u>dilation</u> around the fistula and distal <u>arterial</u> <u>ischemia</u>. The consequences of increased arterial flow in the presence of a congenital AVF are usually <u>hypertrophy</u> and <u>lengthening</u> of the involved extremity. Attention to the lesion may first occur when the child's mother notices a larger extremity. On physical examination, several interesting findings may be noted including

173

1. Dilated superficial veins and varicosities;

2. Venous pulsations;

3. Warmth over the involved area;

4. A palpable thrill over the fistula;

5. A bruit by auscultation;

6. Machinery murmur over the lesion.

The diagnosis is confirmed by arteriography.

The hallmark of these lesions is their tendency to be very extensive, involving a large amount of tissue. Because of this extensive involvement, cure is frequently impossible. Excising these lesions would usually involve amputation or such wide resection that the limb becomes useless. Surgery is usually palliative, done only for complications such as skin breakdown, bleeding, or ulceration. Any surgical procedure on these types of lesions should be done under tourniquet control of the proximal extremity. On some occasions, arterial embolization of the major feeding arterial branches has been successful in obliterating parts of these lesions. The risk of embolization is further necrosis of the skin and tissue overlying the embolized area.

ACQUIRED ARTERIOVENOUS FISTULAE

These lesions are most commonly a result of penetrating trauma to a large adjacent artery and vein that results in a fistulous connection.

Since the blood does not have to cross a capillary bed, the fistula represents the <u>point</u> of <u>lowest</u> <u>systemic</u> <u>vascular</u> resistance within the arterial circuit. This decreased resistance allows large amounts of blood to flow through the fistula, resulting in an <u>increased</u> <u>work</u> <u>load</u> <u>for</u> <u>the</u> <u>heart</u>. The heart compensates by increasing cardiac output and rate. As a result, the natural history of these lesions is progressive enlargement and infection, leading to <u>high</u> <u>output</u> <u>cardiac</u> <u>failure</u>.

Patients may first present in congestive heart failure or may just notice a buzzing sensation over an area of previous trauma. Some patients only notice the dilated varicose veins.

The <u>most</u> <u>impressive</u> <u>physical</u> finding is the <u>Branham's</u> <u>sign</u>, whereby when the fistula <u>is</u> <u>manually</u> compressed and <u>obliterated the</u> pulse decreases. The pulse slows because the <u>peripheral</u> <u>resistance</u> <u>is</u> suddenly increased (blood must now <u>flow</u> <u>across</u> <u>the</u> <u>distal</u> <u>arterial</u> capillary bed as opposed to the fistula), resulting in a <u>rise</u> <u>in</u> <u>blood</u> <u>pressure</u> and a <u>reflex</u> <u>slowing</u> <u>of</u> <u>the</u> <u>pulse</u>. Arteriograms are used to confirm the diagnosis and to plan operative intervention.

Unlike congenital fistulae, these lesions should all be corrected by surgery soon after the diagnosis is made. Surgery involves proximal and distal control of both the artery and vein prior to attacking the lesion. Once the lesion is identified, it is divided, after which both vessels are repaired.

One of the more common acquired arteriovenous fistulas is the AORTIC-CAVAL FISTULA that occurs infrequently in the presence of a large abdominal aortic aneurysm. In these cases, the aorta has eroded into the inferior vena cava. Patients frequently have high output congestive failure with massive leg edema. Surgical repair consists of repair of the fistula from within the aneurysm and then repair of the aneurysm.

SUGGESTED READINGS

1. Flye, M.W., Jordan, B.P., Schwartz, M.Z.: Management of Congenital Malformations. Surgery 94:741-747, 1983.

2. Imparato, A.M., Riles, T.S.: Peripheral Arterial Disease. In Principles of Surgery, edited by S.I. Schwartz, ed 4, pp 931-936. McGraw-Hill, New York, 1984.

3. Johnson, G.: Chronic Traumatic Peripheral Arteriovenous Fistulas. In Vascular Surgery, edited by R.B. Rutherford, ed 1, pp 801-806. W.B. Saunders Co., Philadelphia, 1977.

4. Lindenauer, S.M.: Congenital Arteriovenous Fistula. In Vascular Surgery, edited by R.B. Rutherford, ed 1, pp 793-800. W.B. Saunders Co., Philadelphia, 1977.

5. Rich, N., Spencer, F.C.: Arteriovenous Fistulas. In Vascular Trauma, chapter 9, pp 191-232. W.B. Saunders Co., Philadelphia, 1978.

Chapter 21

Arterial Grafts
with Vascular Disease

The development of biocompatible synthetic arterial substitutes has been one of the most signficant reasons for the rapid development of vascular surgery over the last 30 years. In 1952, Voorhees first reported on the use of Vinyon-N cloth as an arterial substitute. Since then further refinement in manufacturing in conjunction with technical advances in vascular surgery has now made it possible to replace any of the large vessels in the body. Currently, the greatest challenge in graft biomechanics is developing an arterial substitute for vessels less than 4 mm in diameter. As discussed in Chapter 13, the graft of choice at this time for small vessel bypasses and bypasses below the knee remains autogenous vein.

There are three categories of synthetic grafts currently on the market:

1. <u>Dacron</u> in different types of weaves for different uses. The <u>woven Dacron graft</u> is tightly weaved so that there is minimal if any leakage through the wall of the graft. Because of the tighter weave, the graft is less pliable and less expandable. The result is less flexibility of

the graft, which makes it more difficult to sew and maneuver. Woven Dacron grafts are commonly used for abdominal aortic aneurysms and thoracic aortic procedures to minimize blood loss in a situation where the intima that forms within the graft is not of primary concern.

Knitted Dacron is a much looser weave in which the interstices are much wider apart than in the woven pattern. An advantage of the knitted pattern is a more pliable graft that is easier to sew and work with. The other major advantage is the formation of a more extensive pseudointima within the graft as a result of ingrowth into the wider interstices. The graft must be preclotted with the patient's own blood at the time of surgery, to avoid extensive leakage through the graft wall. The preclotting forms a pseudointima within the graft from the patient's own fibrin, which is thought to be important in the long-term patency of the graft in patients with occlusive disease.

A variant of the knitted pattern is the velour knit, in which the loops of yarn in the knitted cloth extend upward at right angles to the surface of the fabric. This imparts a velvet-like feeling to the graft. By using the velour pattern in a knitted graft, the porosity and elasticity of the graft can be adjusted. Double velour grafts have become very popular because they are a mix between a knitted and woven graft, with less leakage than a knitted graft but easier handling characteristics than a woven graft.

2. <u>Polytetrafluoroethylene (PTFE) grafts</u> - The major
manufacturer of the PTFE is the GORETEX Company. GORE-
TEX synthetic grafts are made from synthetic Teflon which
is chemically inert and hydrophilic. GORETEX grafts can
be used in the femoropopliteal position, the aortic
position, or for arteriovenous grafts for hemodialysis.
GORETEX also makes a PTFE suture which is used frequently
with their grafts.   GORETEX also makes thin walled PTFE
(0.4 mm) and thick walled PTFE (0.6 mm) patches to be
used in a variety of clinical situations when patch graft
angioplasty is performed. This includes patching of the
carotid artery during carotid endarterectomy.   The
GORETEX is currently the graft of choice for femoro-
popliteal bypasses above the knee in the absence of
available vein and for arteriovenous grafts for
hemodialysis.

INFECTED ARTERIAL GRAFTS

One of the most dreaded complications in vascular
surgery is infection of a synthetic vascular graft. Grafts
become infected either by direct contamination or by
hematogenous seedings from a distant infection.

Patients with graft infections may first present with
fever of unknown origin or sepsis from an unknown source. On
occasion, patients will present with cellulitis and
induration of the skin over the graft as the first sign.
Physical exam may be remarkable for signs of infection over

an area of the graft. On rare occasion, the patient may have septic emboli distal to the arterial graft. Laboratory values usually reveal an increased white count or possibly an increased erythrocyte sedimentation rate. Isotope-tagged white blood cells from the patient reinjected in conjunction with nuclear medicine scanning have been found to be very effective in documenting graft infections. Patients with intraabdominal sepsis from other sources (i.e., diverticular abscess) may directly seed an intraabdominal graft. Because synthetic grafts are a foreign material, any infection around or near them must be considered to have seeded the graft permanently.

Graft infections in the extremity are a real threat of limb loss, while aortic graft infections are a real threat to the life of the patient. The most important principle in treating a graft infection is <u>removal</u> <u>of</u> <u>all</u> <u>of</u> <u>the</u> <u>infected</u> <u>tissue</u> with <u>removal</u> <u>of</u> <u>the</u> <u>entire</u> <u>synthetic</u> <u>graft</u> that is involved in the process. This usually involves taking out the entire portion of the graft not well incorporated into surrounding tissues. As a result of removal of the graft, distal ischemia frequently occurs.

Management of the subsequent ischemia is a very challenging problem. The sooner the new graft is placed, the greater the risk of it also getting infected. This factor must be weighed against the amount of ischemia the patient can tolerate without risking tissue loss. The optimum treatment is to remove all of the infected tissue and graft, treat the patient with broad spectrum antibiotics I.V. for

7-10 days, and then place the new graft. Unfortunately, in the majority of cases, when the infected graft is removed the resulting ischemia cannot be tolerated without risking some tissue loss. Given this situation the new graft must be placed at the same time as the initial graft is removed.

The second most important concept in treating these patients is that the new graft must be placed in an area that is not infected through clean tissue planes. In patients with aortic graft infections, this usually means an extraanatomical bypass to stay away from the area of infection (see below).

AORTOENTERIC FISTULAE

Aortoenteric fistulae include aortogastric, aorto-colonic, aortointestinal, and most commonly aortoduodenal fistulae. They can be classified as either primary or secondary types. A primary aortoenteric fistula is very rare today and is due to such agents as

1. Tuberculosis, syphilis, or fungus seeding an athero-sclerotic aorta causing erosion between the aorta and gastrointestinal tract;

2. Cancer of the pancreas causing erosion between the aorta and duodenum;

3. Trauma to the duodenum or aorta resulting in a fistulous connection;

4. Radiation treatment causing erosion between the aorta and gastrointestinal tract.

Secondary aortoenteric fistulae are much more common and are usually due to a prosthetic aortic graft. The proximal suture line of an aortic graft lies in direct contact with the duodenum and can erode into the duodenum. The incidence of aortoduodenal fistulae is 0.5-2% in patients with aortic grafts. This complication has been largely circumvented in recent years by keeping the aortic proximal suture line and overlying duodenum out of direct contact. This can be accomplished by closing the aneurysm sac over the proximal anastomosis, placing a Dacron cuff over the proximal anastomosis, closing two layers of retroperitoneal tissue between the duodenum and aorta, or placing omentum between the duodenum and aorta. Essentially any tissue can be used to accomplish the same effect of keeping the duodenum from direct contact with the aorta.

Patients with an aortoenteric fistula present with either upper or lower GI bleeding. Any patient with GI bleeding and an aortic graft in place should be considered to have an aortoenteric fistula until proven otherwise. Frequently these patients present with "herald" bleeding, whereby they bleed a small amount of bright red blood into the upper GI system, stop bleeding, and then hemorrhage massively.

Physical examination is usually unremarkable, as are laboratory values. The diagnosis is made by a high degree of suspicion in patients with the previously mentioned history. If the patient is actively bleeding, upper GI endoscopy may occasionally show blood welling up from the duodenum, but it usually does not reveal the bleeding site. Angiograms are usually not successful in identifying the fistula and are not the test of choice. Currently, the diagnostic test of choice is a CT scan of the abdominal aorta in the area of the duodenum. However CT scans are only helpful if they show an infection around the area of the graft or are suggestive of a communication between the aorta and duodenum. A CT scan does not rule out the diagnosis of an aortoenteric fistula.

Patients who are thought to have an aortoenteric fistula should undergo immediate exploration. If the diagnosis is confirmed, the graft must be considered infected, since the GI contents have been in contact with the graft. Treatment, as in any other graft infection, involves removing the graft in its entirety. The sequence of events for the treatment of aortoenteric fistulae is complicated. Most vascular surgeons agree that if the diagnosis is made and if the patient is stable, then the extraanatomical bypass should be placed first to prevent long periods of ischemia to the lower extremity while the old graft is being removed. Aortoenteric fistulae are very morbid complications with a mortality rate of upwards of 70%.

SUGGESTED READINGS

1. Bunt, T.J.: Synthetic Vascular Graft Infections Clinical Review. Surgery 93:733-745, 1983.

2. Bunt, T.J.: Synthetic Vascular Graft Infections. II. Graft-Enteric Erosions and Graft-Enteric Fistulas. Surgery 94: 1-8, 1983.

3. Champion, M.C., Sullivan, S.N., Coles, J.C., et al.: Aortoenteric Fistula. Ann Surg 195:314-318, 1982.

4. Connolly, J.E., Kwann, J.H., McCart, P.M., et al.: Aortoenteric Fistula. Ann Surg 194:402-412, 1981.

5. Dardik, H., Ibrahim, I., Sussman, B., et al.: Gluteraldehyde-Stabilized Umbilical Vein Prosthesis for Revascularization of the Legs. Am J Surg 138:234-237, 1979.

6. Hanel, K.C., McCabe, M.D., Abbott, W.M., et al.: Current PTFE Grafts: A Biomechanical, Scanning Electron, and Light Microscopic Evaluation. Ann Surg 195:456-463, 1982.

7. Hirsch, S.A., Jarrett, F.: The Use of Stabilized Human Umbilical Vein for Femoralpopliteal Bypass. Ann Surg 200:147-152, 1984.

8. Lindenauer, S.M.: The Synthetic Vascular Prosthesis. In Vascular Surgery, edited by R.B. Rutherford, ed 1, pp 367-379. W.B. Saunders Co., Philadelphia, 1977.

9. Macbeth, G.A., Rubin, J.R., McIntyre, K.E., et al.: The Relevance of Arterial Wall Microbiology to the Treatment of Prosthetic Graft Infections: Graft Infection vs.

Arterial Infection. J Vasc Surg 1:750-756, 1984.

10. Perdue, G.D., Smith, R.B., Ansley, J.D., et al.: Impending Aortoenteric Hemorrhage.: The Effect of Early Recognition on Improved Outcome. Ann Surg 192:237-243, 1980.

11. Weisel, R.D., Johnston, W., Baird, R.J., et al.: Comparison of Conduits for Leg Revascularization. Surgery 89:8-15, 1981.

Chapter 22

Anatomy

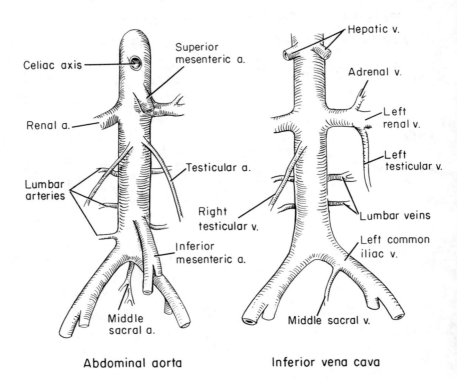

Abdominal aorta   Inferior vena cava

Figure 22.1.   Branches of the abdominal aorta and inferior vena cava.

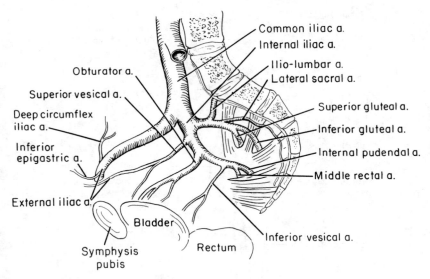

Figure 22.2.   Iliac artery and branches.

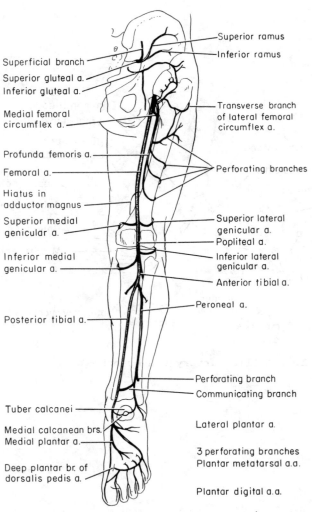

Figure 22.3.   Arteries of the Lower Extremity-Posterior View

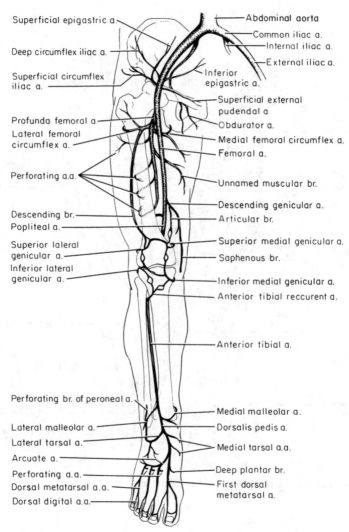

Superficial epigastric a.
Deep circumflex iliac a.
Superficial circumflex iliac a.
Profunda femoral a.
Lateral femoral circumflex a.
Perforating a.a.
Descending br.
Popliteal a.
Superior lateral genicular a.
Inferior lateral genicular a.
Perforating br. of peroneal a.
Lateral malleolar a.
Lateral tarsal a.
Arcuate a.
Perforating a.a.
Dorsal metatarsal a.a.
Dorsal digital a.a.

Abdominal aorta
Common iliac a.
Internal iliac a.
External iliac a.
Inferior epigastric a.
Superficial external pudendal a.
Obdurator a.
Medial femoral circumflex a.
Femoral a.
Unnamed muscular br.
Descending genicular a.
Articular br.
Superior medial genicular a.
Saphenous br.
Inferior medial genicular a.
Anterior tibial reccurent a.
Anterior tibial a.
Medial malleolar a.
Dorsalis pedis a.
Medial tarsal a.a.
Deep plantar br.
First dorsal metatarsal a.

Figure 22.4.   Arteries of the Lower Extremity-Anterior View

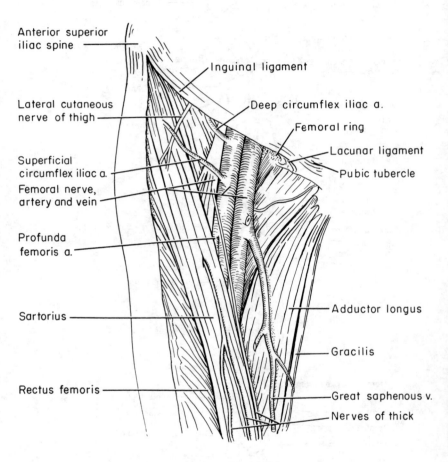

Anterior superior iliac spine

Inguinal ligament

Lateral cutaneous nerve of thigh

Deep circumflex iliac a.

Femoral ring

Lacunar ligament

Superficial circumflex iliac a.

Pubic tubercle

Femoral nerve, artery and vein

Profunda femoris a.

Sartorius

Adductor longus

Gracilis

Rectus femoris

Great saphenous v.

Nerves of thick

Figure 22.5.   Anatomy of the inguinal region.

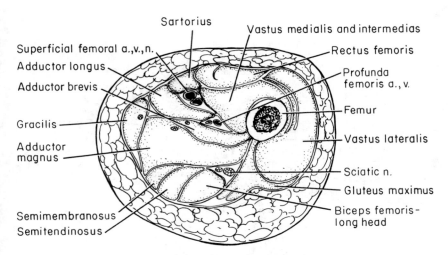

Sartorius

Vastus medialis and intermedias

Superficial femoral a.,v.,n.

Rectus femoris

Adductor longus

Profunda femoris a., v.

Adductor brevis

Femur

Gracilis

Vastus lateralis

Adductor magnus

Sciatic n.

Gluteus maximus

Semimembranosus

Biceps femoris-long head

Semitendinosus

Cross section of thigh (middle)

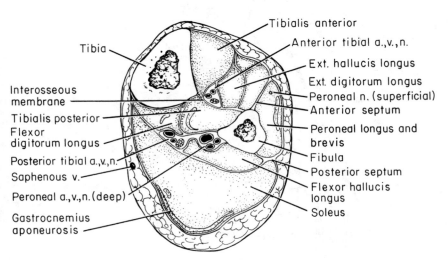

Tibialis anterior

Tibia

Anterior tibial a.,v.,n.

Ext. hallucis longus

Interosseous membrane

Ext. digitorum longus

Peroneal n. (superficial)

Tibialis posterior

Anterior septum

Flexor digitorum longus

Peroneal longus and brevis

Posterior tibial a.,v.,n.

Fibula

Saphenous v.

Posterior septum

Peroneal a.,v.,n.(deep)

Flexor hallucis longus

Gastrocnemius aponeurosis

Soleus

Figure 22.6.   Cross-section of the leg.

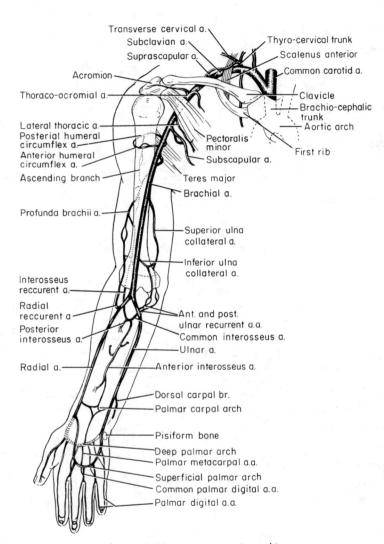

Figure 22.7.   Arteries of the upper extremity.

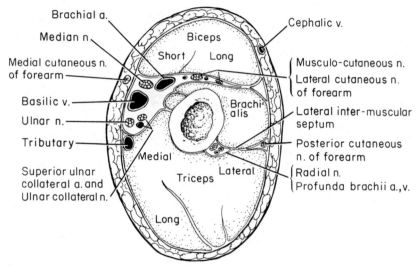

Figure 22.8.   Cross-section of the arm.